# Pain Management

## How to Improve Your Life With Biohacks

*(Learn How to Use Herbs to Alleviate Chronic and Acute Pain and Inflammation)*

**Ross Merrick**

Published By **Elena Holly**

# Ross Merrick

*Pain Management: How to Improve Your Life With Biohacks (Learn How to Use Herbs to Alleviate Chronic and Acute Pain and Inflammation)*

**ISBN 978-1-998038-26-8**

No part of this guidebook shall be reproduced in any form without permission in writing from the publisher except in the case of brief quotations embodied in critical articles or reviews.

Legal & Disclaimer

Table Of Contents

# Chapter 1: Pain, Pain ... Why Won't It Go Away?

I recall Joan, who changed into adamant she had no longer had any injuries or accidents however were dealing with sciatic pain down the back of her proper leg for almost two a long term. This pain had not resolved after endless remedies in pretty plenty each ache profession you can think about, which embody rub down remedy, chiropractic and bodily remedy, and orthopedic treatments. Testing observed out now not some thing incorrect, and he or she or he suspected that the doctors concept she changed into making it up. No one understood why she had this ache that wouldn't depart.

Pain is a topic that may be referred to, debated, and researched until the end of time because technological expertise constantly learns greater about it. What have become believed about pain as quickly as I changed into in college is alas vintage.

Reams were written about this difficulty remember, and this single financial catastrophe will most sincerely no longer cowl even a tiny part of all the tremendous records. My intention is to offer a easy knowledge of what's currently stated and what I have seen for the motive that 1994 as a physical therapist. My purpose is this financial ruin will assist you type out which path to take and may even help you decrease your ache.

Your ache may be silly, sharp, taking pictures, burning, extreme, aching, tingling, throbbing, or nagging. It may be intermittent or constant. It may additionally moreover increase or decrease in intensity all through the day or night. Your ache can also rise up specifically positions or take place at the same time as you're changing positions, like going from sitting to fame. It may moreover seem in case you take a seat down down too prolonged, stand too long, or walk too lengthy. Too prolonged may be as low as three minutes. Your ache can be worse at night time time when you are trying to sleep, or worse inside the morning whilst you awaken.

Pain may be considerably one-of-a-type amongst  humans of the same age, the equal gender, the same career, the identical health degree, and with the identical prognosis. This is the precept reason treating pain successfully is so tough. You can't diagnose a person's pain from a e-book like you could a illness method: there are too many variables.

Some (not generally identified) Reasons Pain Doesn't Go Away

The aspect of this chapter is to talk about why ache takes location with out apparent coincidence or harm, and why ache doesn't leave as soon as the offending stimuli have ceased (like at the same time as you fall from a ladder and hit your knee). In the case of a fall, the impact creates pain inside the

2d, however if there can be no harm to the joint (say, knee), which embody a fracture or torn ligament, why does the knee although hurt months later? Even if a number one damage takes location, why does it although harm after recovery seems to be entire? Worse but, what if there was no damage or fall however your knee clearly began out hurting for no obvious cause?

The many misconceptions about pain can lead human beings on a wild goose chase to clear up it without success. Often, the motives aren't obvious or well understood, so let's start with what I certainly have positioned to be one of the maximum commonplace reasons for pain: a loss of characteristic in one of the 3 planes of motion.

1. Pain and Three-Plane Function

Your frame is designed to move in all 3 planes of movement and to control that motion with no trouble in the course of bodily pastime. You skip beforehand and back or side to aspect, and you switch right and left. If you lack movement in any person or extra of these three planes, ache is the cease end result. If you lack balance in any of these 3 planes, pain is the cease end end result. Pain can occur in areas a long manner far from any joint that lacks any of those motions.

If your hip lacks rotation, or your ankle lacks dorsiflexion, your knee will now not be a glad camper. If you have were given were given pain or restricted movement while turning your hip, this may have an effect on your knee. If you have pain or confined motion at the same time as you bend your ankle and lift your ft upward, your knee may be affected. It is crucial to repair three-plane function to your hip and ankle, if this is in which the offender lies, at the way to effectively treatment knee ache. You can deal with your knee (the sufferer) until the cows come domestic, however until you address the hip issue or ankle problem (the wrongdoer), your knee ache will now not see eternal choice. The bankruptcy on knee pain teaches you more approximately this.

Many humans in pain are chasing the signs of their pain. They are first-class treating the sufferers which may be being "beat up" by way of the usage of the perpetrator, it is the actual motive you have got were given pain. This reality is why I evolved the Move Without Pain software program application, which teaches you what has most effective been taught to movement and healthcare experts and experts till now. You can learn how to repair three-plane feature and efficiently do away with pain from your frame with this application. More element approximately this training is in Part three, and the useful resource section will offer you with get admission to to a unfastened online recorded beauty to evaluate your very personal 3-plane characteristic in most effective 24 minutes. There is also a unfastened elegance that teaches a manner to train your body and repair three-aircraft feature. Many humans have removed persistent pain because of this unfastened elegance!

2. Pain and Biomechanics Gone Awry

If you have got persistent ache that is not going away, it may be you sustained an damage years in the past from a fall or twist of fate you've got have been given forgotten or don't assume may want to have some element to do together with your contemporary signs and symptoms. I beg to vary.

If you ever sprained an ankle stepping off a decrease, your ankle fashion of movement and function may be affected long after the damage. Remember John and his neck pain? Or you can have picked up a suitcase that have become an lousy lot heavier than anticipated. Or you'll probably have been at a prevent light together together with your foot on the brake and rear-ended, which created a biomechanical problem along side your sacrum or spine. You may additionally have had an trouble for quite some time with out knowing it, but your body has been compensating to permit you to hold to feature as typically as viable. Then within the future (or night time time), pain began out. It regarded to start for no suitable purpose. You don't keep in mind a present day damage or twist of future, but your shoulder, or knee, or hip, or lower lower back just started out out to harm.

The extraordinary records is manual techniques and self-care strategies described in Part 3 can address the ones issues pretty successfully.

three. Pain and Fascial Injury

What many people are not aware about is that clearly sitting for prolonged intervals can impair your fascia and bring about compression and damage of the cells. Fascia is that milky-searching saranwrap-like stuff that exists amongst your pores and skin and your muscles. Think of a piece of raw chook and look some of the pores and pores and skin and the pork. You will see it there. Fascia exists quite plenty everywhere in your frame. If you stiffen on the identical time as you sit down down down for a while and struggle to upward push up at once, it is able to be compressed fascia. If you are not able to region flat to your over again without ache, an impaired and inefficient fascial system may be your problem.

Another manner your fascia becomes impaired is whilst it is lessen through, whether or not or no longer or not from surgery or an harm. This wonderful tissue has a wonderfully clean gliding ground while working the manner it became designed, however it adheres to structures whilst it's miles lessen through. I had a affected man or woman injured thru way of a heavy steel door being opened tough into her arm. Her shoulder ache remained so excessive she struggled to install writing down on her sufferers' charts for numerous weeks. She moreover had a deep scar from  C-sections and an stomach surgical treatment. I taught her a fascial method to release the scar, and she turned into blown away by means of how loads an awful lot less complex it turn out to be to get up straighter and through the multiplied period in her stride even as walking. She additionally had plenty less pain from the harm to her shoulder! The impaired gliding capacity of her fascia became inhibiting recuperation in her shoulder vicinity because it affected freedom of movement. (I truly have supplied statistics about a great video in Resources that shows a way to launch a scar.)

Whether from surgical treatment or damage, scar tissue can substantially limit motion, inhibit healing, and have an impact on characteristic everywhere on your frame, essential to chronic ache. You may be doing all of the right topics: exercising efficaciously, stretching, and strengthening, however nonetheless have chronic pain regions on your body. If this is the case, your fascial machine may be the culprit, because of the fact that your fascia does not stretch like a muscle. It does not reply to strengthening or normal motion physical sports activities. Your fascial device requires specific mechanical pressures to stimulate fluid production, rehydrate the tool, and alleviate compression.

There is a proper way and a wrong way to cope with your fascial device. Ironing your frame like a blouse with a hard foam roller is the incorrect way! The suitable facts is that you could honestly repair fitness to this device, and the adjustments can upward thrust up at once. Lying flat to your decrease again can be snug all another time! I even have taught loads of humans inside the health facility, in non-public video consultations, and in commands on the network college, a manner to self-deal with their fascia. Many have received comfort from pain and pain in as little as ten mins. It works! More facts about this method is in Part three.

4. Pain and Chronic Imbalances

You can be any such individuals who say, "my whole left facet is tousled" or "all my pain is on my proper facet." Imbalance can manifest at the same time as your body doesn't play exquisite from one element to the alternative or some of your muscle tissues don't carry out as designed in remarkable regions of the body. When each of these things happens, chronic pain is regularly the end result.

An imbalance can arise even as you require a specific frame detail to artwork a excessive best way for an prolonged length. One instance might be a affected person I had who drove a forklift in opposite for maximum of his going for walks hours while grew to come to be to the right searching behind him. Another example is probably if you sit down down hunched beforehand at a desk all day.

Imagine exercising these joints in an try and "recuperation" the hassle. You only come to be risking more damage. There is a self-care method in Part three that works to remedy imbalances over 80% of the time, regularly the number one time you operate it.

5. Pain and Impaired Circulation

You might be surprised to discover that one of the most commonplace causes of once more pain is not tested in a clinical medical doctor's administrative center. While there may be a couple of motive for another time pain, impaired circulate can be a considerable contributing trouble. Your body has many miles of blood vessels, and all of them matter wide variety. There has been a focus for decades on go with the flow to your coronary coronary coronary heart and your thoughts, but what approximately your backbone?

You have heard the time period cardiovascular disorder (CVD) but have you ever heard about lumbar artery ailment? (I apprehend, not a few different illness!) The truth is they may be every due to the same issue. Blood vessels don't discriminate close to harm and impairment. If you have problems together along with your circulate anywhere, you have it everywhere, and reduced glide to the spine has examined to correlate to lower back ache, degenerative disc sickness, sciatic ache, deep hip ache with exercise, and additional.

Dr. Lena Kauppila has posted massive studies approximately the connection among CVD and again pain. Her art work suggests how impaired lumbar circulate correlates to ache and extreme issues which have been blamed on surely "growing older" through manner of healthcare specialists. (I percentage some of her numerous research within the financial disaster on again pain.)

The backside line is that once the lumbar arteries are blocked by means of manner of way of calcifications and plaques, they're no longer imparting the healthful blood supply important to the spine, ensuing in ailment, disc ailment, bone sickness, and ache.

When now not some thing indicates up on MRIs or X-rays that explains the persistent lower back ache, is truely anyone trying out lumbar artery feature? Is absolutely everyone contemplating the pain as a possible impaired go with the go with the flow hassle? The standard route for persistent lower back ache that does not clear up is from doctor to orthopedist to pain manage, yet all of the ache manipulate remedies inside the global will no longer paintings if your backbone isn't always getting the right blood deliver.

6. Pain and Chronic Inflammation

Chronic infection is profoundly related to chronic ache situations. If your body is experiencing continual contamination, the give up give up result can be pain inside the course of, or moderate to severe ache in positive joints. Diagnoses like fibromyalgia strongly correlate with high tiers of infection.[1, 2] Another aspect that correlates with immoderate tiers of infection to your body? Food! You will studies more in Part 3, this is right data as it way you may restore yourself!

Carrying extra weight is also correlated to persistent inflammation within the clinical literature. Excess body weight technique advanced frame fat, and fat cells promote inflammatory mechanisms in the frame.[3] Inflammatory cytokines in excess can bring about infection and tissue damage. This contributing element approach more weight promotes infection for your body.

While weight loss is seen to reduce contamination and ache, one of the first topics I hear even as training my beauty, Nourish Away Pain for Lifelong Wellbeing, at the local people college is that pain is considerably reduced or long lengthy beyond in as low as one week! This technique you don't constantly want to take a look at for weight reduction to take vicinity in advance than you experience better. Just converting the way you nourish your frame can rework the manner you feel. The Resources section shares records about a loose PDF download with greater records.

7. Pain, Stress, and Trauma

An emotional harm from beyond activities, or a lifestyles full of overwhelming responsibility, can result in persistent pain problems. Indeed, the American Institute of Stress reviews seventy five% to 90% of visits to primary care physicians end result from stress-related troubles. If you recall, maximum healthcare visits are for ache, but

17

why must stress create infection or pain? It's due to the chemical cascade that your mind and emotions create. I will try to simplify the complex chemistry worried.

Let's begin with the chemical cascade that takes location with a perception, greater in particular an emotional idea, like worry. Since fear is a common emotion for masses humans, it's critical you recognize the manner it impacts your frame chemically and, ultimately, chronically. Everyday troubles, like now not having enough cash to pay the payments, being overdue for paintings due to web site traffic or weather, or being involved about your youngsters's safety in school or daycare, can instill a normal, low degree of worry on your frame. This fear sign is relayed for your brain (thalamus > amygdala), which releases neurotransmitters for the duration of your body—drastically glutamate, it truly is, basically, the chemical inside the lower back of worry. Your mind has three conventional responses to fear: walking, preventing, and freezing. This is the combat or flight response, but a greater correct time period is the combat, flight, or freeze reaction. Ever had a nightmare in that you had been frozen with fear?

Your hypothalamus controls the ones responses thru increased coronary heart fee and different functions. Your adrenal glands then signal to send out cortisol and adrenaline, and glucose is then released into your bloodstream to provide energy to run or combat as desired. Now do not forget you are sitting at your table and you have were given have been given closing dates you're afraid you acquired't meet, or your boss is tough to deal with and you're worried you can lose your venture. Those thoughts and emotions of fear additionally elicit a chemical response to your frame. Imagine you have got got have been given two video video games and 3 practices you need to get your youngsters to this week and despite the fact that cope with food, assist with homework, domestic responsibilities, laundry, and so forth. While you are in a constant kingdom of low-diploma worry that you received't get all of it completed, your frame is constantly freeing these chemical materials. Don't you determined your muscle tissue is probably prepared to combat or flight or freeze on a in no way-completing foundation? This regular anxiety results in pain.

Memories of trauma or abuse purpose the identical chemical reaction from the emotion that passed off sooner or later of the trauma. Your frame believes it's far in risk the immediate the ones reminiscences occur, even if the occasion passed off years ago. There is likewise some aspect referred to as a 'motive' that can carry upon those emotions and chemical responses without warning. When you examine or listen or fragrance some thing that reminds your body of the equal hazard it changed into in even as the trauma to start with happened, chemical launch takes place. Let me provide some examples.

If you professional a fall or accident at the equal time as a song changed into gambling and also you hear the music years later, this could motive a chemical release. Or say you expert abuse through someone who wore a selected cologne, and now you heady scent that cologne. Your frame can even undergo in thoughts the position it grow to be in even as the ache or damage came about (like sitting inside the automobile at the equal time as rear-ended) and now your frame does it's remarkable to preserve you out of that role so that you received't be injured over again.

Thankfully, there is a way to retrain your thoughts just so the recollections do not cause the feelings and the resultant chemical cascade. The artwork of Dr. John Sarno, Dr. Jonathon Kuttner, and Dr.

Caroline Leaf additionally let you (see Resources).

I absolutely have co-led a help organization for the reason that 1999 for ladies who have been abused. I really have visible, up near and personal, the consequences of emotional, intellectual, sexual, and physical trauma. I simply have furthermore visible limitless girls let loose and lead healthful, happy lives. When issues are buried and no longer addressed in a way that brings recovery, they'll be buried alive. If you have got got a information of trauma, this will be part of the cause your ache is not going away. There are more information about this group determined at cameo.Gracefellowship.Com.

eight. Pain and Altered Perception

The foundation of changing ache notion is a subject that's quite complex and now not however clearly understood. Essentially, electrically or medically stimulating specific areas of your mind can regulate ache. This stimulation is how opioids artwork. You have pain-modulating pathways for your mind that, whilst inspired, manage the interest of the information coming out of your nociceptors (ache nerve cells).

Let me provide a smooth example of modulating ache. When you hit your shin, your first instinct is to rub it vigorously for a minute or . You do that to lessen the feeling of sharp pain by means of way of activating nerve cells focusing on reporting stress. By rubbing your leg, you are stimulating your thoughts to provide ache consolation.

The problem starts offevolved at the same time as those pain-modulating pathways emerge as faulty and intense ache isn't dealt with within the normal way. Hyperalgesia and allodynia are such faults. Hyperalgesia is at the equal time as your body over responds to stimulus and develops an prolonged sensitivity to ache. What would possibly were the mildest of pain in advance than is felt as severe ache. An example is transferring a joint this is enhancing from a slight sprain. Mild ache is regular; severe pain isn't always.

Allodynia is at the same time as pain occurs in reaction to a stimulus that is not normally considered noxious, like a mild breeze. I in reality have visible patients broaden allodynia from injuries (falls, vehicle accidents) that should have healed in only some weeks. I consider going for walks with a candy female who slipped on her porch and sprained her ankle. She changed into now not succesful to walk on that foot for months due to excessive ache. The harm itself modified into no longer extreme; but weeks later, she could not even tolerate a fan blowing air on her foot because it changed into too painful. We were able to work alongside facet her and desensitize the ones nociceptors, however it took some time.

Let me permit you to know the relaxation of Joan's story.

When I assessed Joan's pelvis, I placed a sacral torsion, it truly is even as the sacrum doesn't line up correctly with the hip bones. When this takes place, a small muscle referred to as the "piriformis" can spasm due to the truth it's miles being pulled abnormally. This muscle, even as in spasm, can get worse the sciatic nerve and create ache in the butt or down the leg. We corrected the torsion and then labored on getting the piriformis muscle to launch.

It took a few doing, however at the same time as her piriformis in the end launched, she  remembered an occasion that took place twenty years formerly. She have been setting garments on a clothesline at the pinnacle of the stairs on her decrease lower back porch and slipped on the morning dew and fell down the steps. She had forgotten it till the discharge of her piriformis introduced on her recollection. I will in no manner overlook her crying out even as she felt warm temperature down her leg to her ankle because the muscle released.

We have covered plenty, however here's a summary of reasons for why ache doesn't leave and some questions to ask yourself.

- 

Impaired practical mobility and balance: Are your important body components loading well to offer and control motion in all 3 planes of motion?

- 

Biomechanics lengthy beyond awry: Are your joints aligned efficiently?

- 

Dehydrated/compressed fascia: Do you're taking a seat all the time? Do you have scars?

-

Chronic imbalance: Is one factor of your frame strolling in every other manner than the opportunity thing?

- 

Impaired flow: Are your cells getting the oxygen and vitamins they need?

- 

Chronic inflammation: Are you selling contamination in your frame via your weight loss plan?

- 

Psychological/emotional trauma and strain: Have you skilled past trauma or are you currently overwhelmed?

- 

Pain notion lengthy long beyond awry: Do you appear to have signs and signs and symptoms of hyperalgesia, allodynia, or wonderful ache patterns?

## Chapter 2: Meds, Treatments, Procedures, And Other Bad Ideas

Meet Joe, who dreams he'd had the information earlier than agreeing to a prescribed medicinal drug. He had intense pain due to injuries from a car twist of fate, ache that started out in his lower returned and moved to his testicles. They had no idea why he had this pain and had not completed an MRI to locate the possible cause. Nevertheless, in excruciating ache, he underwent a nerve block device. This remedy changed into a literal and figurative shot in the dark and best faded his ache slightly for approximately 3 days. Then the ache decrease again with a vengeance. He end up then prescribed gabapentin to deal with the ache. They though had no concept why he had this pain. You acquired't take shipping of as real with what occurred to Joe ...

The maximum critical questions to ask even as you're recommended to start a remedy, take a take a look at, or go through a way are: How a bargain damage will it do? And how lots help will or not it's with my hassle?

With solutions to the ones questions, you could make up your non-public thoughts, really informed, and pick out what's first-rate for you. You may be questioning which you aren't a clinical health practitioner, so how are you going to understand the information and make a clever desire? Let me positioned this in attitude for you. You are in all likelihood now not a mechanic, but you are capable of make an informed choice about looking for a automobile. You do your research and ask questions. You are possibly no longer a contractor, plumber, electrician, or wooden employee, however you could make an informed choice about looking for a home.

Similarly, you do now not want to be a medical doctor or medical professional to make a realistic choice approximately your healthcare options. You virtually want honest statistics about what is being recommended and make better choices for progressed fitness outcomes. How well does it work, and what are the dangers and side consequences? Spoiler alert! Many pain drugs are often ineffective and function severa dangerous factor results.

You should recognize the information so that you could make better alternatives for stepped forward effects concerning your health.

Pain Medications: Do they artwork and are the side consequences well worth it?

Before I hold, an essential word: I do now not propose everyone to stop prescribed or encouraged drug treatments. I educate each client about all recognised risks and benefits and urge humans to speak with their prescribing practitioner earlier than making any changes, as some pills are risky to prevent and function excessive withdrawal problems. Always consult an expert in advance than stopping any prescribed remedy.

That stated, it's essential to realise that scientific professionals have four medication options to prescribe for the remedy of ache:

- 

Analgesics

- 

Anti-inflammatories

- 

Opioids

- 

Antidepressants

Analgesics (Acetaminophen)

Typically, the number one advice given to a person who comes to the medical doctor with a criticism of pain is to take an anti-inflammatory or analgesic (ache) remedy.

Acetaminophen is the maximum commonplace due to the fact it's miles taken into consideration an entire lot less risky on your digestive tract than NSAIDs. The most famous shape of acetaminophen is Tylenol.

Does it art work for pain? Not sincerely.

Studies show acetaminophen is useless for low decrease again pain (every acute and continual) and nearly vain for osteoarthritic ache and anxiety headache.

- 

 Low once more pain trials display no pain comfort, no advanced healing tempo, and no amazing effect with any trouble (disability, feature, notable of life, or high-quality of sleep). Yet, this remedy is the primary-line scientific remedy for another time ache.1

-

Osteoarthritis ache studies pronounced a 4% ache cut price.2 Physical characteristic and stiffness have been considered approximately the identical among the drugs and the placebo.

- 

Tension-kind headache ache studies confirmed only a five% effectiveness in ache treatment.three

One wouldn't thoughts the low expenses of effectiveness if there have been no dangers worried with its use, but this is not the case. Acetaminophen toxicity is pretty extreme and may rise up without warning, as it's miles presently an issue in over six hundred pills (every over-the-counter and pharmaceuticals). When taken on my own, there's a small margin a number of the encouraged maximum dosage and overdose, and at the same time as taken for pain alongside issue different medicines, toxicity will become a extreme risk.

Acetaminophen overdose sends round fifty nine,000 Americans to the emergency room annually and effects in 38,000 hospitalizations a 12 months.four

In small portions, this drug is detoxified by using the use of your liver and excreted out of your frame. But in huge portions or in fitness-compromised humans, it overwhelms the cleansing device and begins offevolved offevolved destroying liver tissue. This drug does now not come without substantial risks for your fitness while consumed often. My dad died at the age of ninety 3. He have become yellow some days earlier than he exceeded due to the fact his liver could not detoxify the acetaminophen he have become given each day for joint ache. I don't maintain all people answerable for his dying, as he was notably sick with persistent lymphocytic leukemia at the surrender of his lengthy life, however I do consider the acetaminophen may additionally have hastened his lack of life.

Non-Steroidal Anti-Inflammatory Drugs (NSAIDs)

If your hassle is because of contamination, acetaminophen will no longer assist with that, so NSAIDs are advocated. NSAIDs are generally recommended for pain, specifically if it consists of infection from an harm, contamination, illness method (e.G., arthritis), or a surgical treatment.

There are selective and non-selective NSAIDs. Selective NSAIDs (cox-2 inhibitors) are touted to be heaps much less disturbing to your gastrointestinal tract than non-selective kinds. Conventional non-selective NSAIDs are aspirin, ibuprofen (e.G., Advil, Motrin, Midol), and naproxen (e.G., Aleve, Naprosyn). The best selective NSAID currently to be had within the United States is Celebrex. Two different manufacturers, Vioxx and Bextra, have been withdrawn from the market in 2004 and 2005 respectively, because of the truth they excessively elevated the chance of heart assaults and strokes with lengthy-term use. In one of a kind terms, human beings have been in particular demise while the use of those drugs. This is a clear case of threat outweighing advantage!

Do NSAIDs art work for pain? Looking at the proof to guide using NSAIDs for spinal ache, neuropathic ache, knee pain, and placed up-operative pain, the effects are a good deal lots less than excellent. I will percent a few records and permit you make a decision for yourself.

•35 decrease lower back pain studies located that for every affected person who recommended a clinically tremendous lower in ache after  weeks on an NSAID, every one-of-a-kind six did no longer.five

•No legitimate evidence exists whether or now not NSAIDs artwork or not for neuropathic pain.6

•Knee pain: "NSAIDs can lessen brief time period pain in osteoarthritis of the knee barely better than placebo, however the modern-day assessment does not help extended-time period use of NSAIDs for this situation. As critical negative outcomes are associated with oral NSAIDs, only restrained use may be advocated."7

•In acute postoperative ache, nine studies stated some advantage in treating ache with NSAIDs.eight When treating 27 human beings, ten had at the least 50% comfort of ache. Aspirin use for acute postoperative ache produced a similar stop end result. Seventy- randomized single-dose trials confirmed one in 4 acquired 50% ache treatment, but not without risks.9 "Drowsiness and gastric inflammation have been seen as big damaging outcomes in spite of the truth that the research have been unmarried-dose. This manner lengthy-term use includes critical dangers."

Side results of prolonged-term use are belly infection, ulcers, heartburn, diarrhea, fluid retention, kidney ailment, and cardiovascular disorder.10 Yes, cardiovascular disease is related to NSAID use! Over 22,000 research document numerous fitness risks of the use of NSAIDs.eleven

Since NSAID use is associated with over sixteen,000 annual gastrointestinal bleeding-associated deaths and accelerated risk of high-quality cardiac troubles, like atrial traumatic infection, the dangers seem to an extended manner outweigh the benefits.12-14 I don't keep in mind truly definitely anybody wants to harm their coronary heart or their digestive device while searching for to solve their ache.

Opioids

Opioid use has emerge as a lethal problem. Not exceptional does it convey a immoderate addiction risk, however all-reason mortality extensively will growth whilst in evaluation with non-selective NSAID use.

Most humans believe that opioids are the most amazing ache relievers, yet this isn't always accurate. Taking acetaminophen and ibuprofen together is seen to be identical to or more powerful in treating submit-operative ache than opioids!15-17

How well do opioids paintings for pain and what harm to health is visible from their use? Looking at continual low lower back ache indicates handiest quick-time period comfort, without a proof of prolonged-term effectiveness.18 In half of of those trials, as a minimum 50% of people forestall the trial because of the reality the facet results outweighed the advantages, or the medication didn't artwork the least bit. Why then are we able to anticipate opioids are an superb idea for treating continual pain if it is not the most robust ache treatment and no evidence exists to assist long-term use (greater than 4 months) to deal with persistent pain?

Ultracet is a aggregate remedy, inclusive of the opioid tramadol and acetaminophen, and it's far visible to lower ache thru best round 15% with the doubtful factor effects of nausea, dizziness, and constipation.19 Is a 15% good deal in pain really worth those facet results?

Opioids moreover purpose respiration misery and absence of life whilst taken in excessive doses or on the same time as combined with distinct substances, specially alcohol. I had a relative die at the same time as mendacity on her dwelling room sofa. She had persistent again pain for years and feature grow to be taking ache medicinal drugs regularly, and she or he or he or he surely stopped respiration. She emerge as a splendid, loving female in her forties with a husband and children who have been devastated by the use of her loss.

If a person turns into unresponsive, and is respiratory shallowly and has blue lips and nail beds, they ought to get emergency remedy proper away. Naloxone works to dam the receptors from the opioids, and naloxone kits are made to be had in an try to maintain lives. I supply one in my bag. Please see Resources for extra data.

Sadly, regardless of a six hundred% increase in the use of opioids within the remaining a long time inside the U.S., persistent pain has no longer decreased.20 Americans suffered as lots incapacity from yet again and neck ache in 2010 as they did in 1990, earlier than the escalation inside the prescribing of opioids.21 It is presently predicted that greater than 9 million Americans use opioids for the treatment of persistent nonmalignant pain but it's now not running: Americans are despite the fact that in pain.22 A massive test confirmed human beings with chronic pain who've been on chronic opioid therapy (COT) had higher degrees of ache, poorer exceptional of life, and had been less practical than people with persistent ache who were no longer on COT.23 Clearly, opioids aren't the solution to pain that doesn't leave.

Antidepressants

Medications prescribed for despair have come to be extensively used in pain remedy, however the truth that their effectiveness is stated to be pretty confined. A take a look at searching at antidepressants and ache shows that antidepressants have an analgesic impact, but how those pills work for pain is not referred to.24 Is this sound technological understanding?

Study effects looking at duloxetine (provided as Cymbalta) for treating painful diabetic neuropathy, fibromyalgia, painful physical signs and signs, and crucial neuropathic ache are much less than dazzling considering the high dangers worried:25

•a hundred subjects had to be treated for 18 of the topics to experience a 50% discount in ache.

•Fibromyalgia and depressive ache saw thirteen out of 100 reporting 50% discount in ache with remedy.

•No impact changed into observed to arise on the same time as treating fundamental neuropathic pain.

I recall a affected individual with a piece-associated again harm, a herniated disc, which stored him from being capable of paintings. He end up a in reality outstanding guy, the sort of character you would really like to have as a neighbor, who cherished his family and in reality wanted to get again to art work and resume his life. His medical doctor prescribed an antidepressant to cope with his pain. The guy shared with me that he had most effective been taking it for three days and have become experiencing seriously disturbing nightmares, similarly to different frightening aspect outcomes. He come to be visibly shaken with the aid of the use of using this. While it's miles out of doors the scope of my practice to advocate everyone concerning the taking of prescribed drug remedies, I am ethically fine to ensure my patients are nicely knowledgeable, so I confirmed him the literature concerning the aspect effects of this medication. His first query modified into, "Where are the advantages?" His pain come to be not reduced, and he changed into though out of hard work. His medical doctor had now not informed him of the dangers of taking this remedy. He selected to speak to his clinical health practitioner and save you the medication. His ache grow to be then managed with a TENS unit (no element consequences), and his disc problem persisted to heal and decorate over the years. A TENS unit is a small device that gives slight electric powered stimulation that overrides the pain message and blocks it from being acquired by using way of the mind.

The remaining and maximum critical truth concerning the dangers of using this beauty of medication is that this: The U.S. Food and Drug Administration (FDA) issued a drug safety alert on extended suicidal conduct with antidepressants in July 2005 and a drug safety alert on most vital congenital malformations in September 2005.26 In the scientific global, the worry of a contemporary mom harming herself or her baby due to positioned up-partum depression has outweighed any risks of harming the toddler in some unspecified time in the future of pregnancy.

Joe, whom you met on the start of the chapter, changed into now not well knowledgeable of the dangers of his prescribed remedy. Let's go lower back now to his story.

Joe professional extreme element outcomes from the gabapentin, together with rash, intense fatigue, and reminiscence loss. Since his ache emerge as however slight to immoderate, he modified into counseled with the beneficial aid of his medical doctor to double the dosage, regardless of his side effects at the modern-day dosage! He ended up within the ER with acute chest pain and modified into identified with angina. One of the severa facet outcomes of gabapentin is myocardial infarction, AKA coronary coronary heart assault.27

Joe modified into in no way informed of those dangers, and no one of a kind alternatives were given to cope with his pain. I changed into asked by using way of Joe's physical therapist to are searching for advice from in this case. I used advanced pressure and counterstrain techniques, which supplied short moments of 0 (out of ten) ache for the number one time considering the reality that his twist of fate.

There aren't any component consequences of this slight method!

Since I changed into only asked to seek recommendation from in this situation and was not his number one clinician, I don't understand how Joe ended up. Last I knew, he grow to be looking in advance to approval from Workers Compensation for an MRI because of the fact his accident occurred in a chunk vehicle (he became not the the usage of force).

I determined this declaration currently on webmd.Com: "If your clinical physician has directed you to use this product, remember that he or she has judged that the benefit to you is greater than the risk of side effects." Do you actually need a person other than your self identifying which dangers are accurate enough to enjoy? You ought to be knowledgeable!

Common Medical Treatments for Pain: Do they art work? Are they secure?

Some radical techniques arise within the ache management international, which includes destroying nerves with warmness, surgically implanting nerve stimulators, and fusing spinal segments. Many of these procedures are achieved so regularly they may be taken into consideration common, so now looks as if a excellent time to tell you of a take a look at that indicates doing now not some issue the least bit for acute returned pain can be a terrific concept, because of the fact pain is visible to clear up without intervention more than 1/2 of the time.28 However, for the reason that doing not anything is not regularly desired as an preference by using the usage of someone in pain, right proper here are the commonly performed treatments.

Nerve Blocks/Steroid Injections

Before you settle to an injection on your back or neck, recognise that any use of steroids for spinal injection is not FDA legal and brought into attention "off label" use.

In 2014, the FDA warned injection of corticosteroids into the epidural vicinity of the spine must bring about unusual however excessive neurological sports, which includes "loss of imaginative and prescient, stroke, paralysis, and shortage of life."29 Indeed, in 2012–13, a virulent disease of fungal meningitis because of inflamed steroids uncovered as many as 13,000 sufferers country wide, ensuing in 751 meningitis infections and at the least sixty four deaths.30

Let's see if those risks are outweighed via the blessings.

Epidural steroid injections are regularly given to deal with low again and sciatica pain. Pain relief, if it takes vicinity in any respect, has an inclination to be short, and injections aren't advised for prolonged-time period use. A National Institute of Health-funded have a examine confirmed prolonged-time period results were worse among those who acquired the injections, in comparison with those who did now not. Repeated use of those injections is established to growth sensible impairment, this is in no manner a person's intention even as seeking out remedy for pain.

Lumbar factor joint injection has a excessive technical failure rate due to the truth the motive is omitted with the aid of manner of the expert nearly 40% of the time.31 This is a dark failure price for the second one maximum usually finished approach for persistent pain; plus the proof that they art work well is not supported inside the studies.32 Most literature opinions file injections for again ache are vain.32-36

Corticosteroid injections are usually used to cope with pain in areas apart from the spine, together with shoulders, elbows, hips, and knees. Are they powerful? Let's see.

Manual physical remedy  times a week for 3 weeks became visible as effective as up to three corticosteroid injections during a one-one year observe up of subjects with shoulder impingement syndrome.37 But, the injection company visited greater physicians/healthcare experts and had more procedures than the manual physical treatment (PT) organisation. You are higher off with six PT visits, for the reason that injections have the threat of dying of nearby bone (osteonecrosis), bone infection (osteomyelitis), nerve damage, deterioration of cartilage, tendon weakening or rupture, and thinning of the adjacent bone (osteoporosis).38,39

I even have come to be requested to seek advice from an elderly woman, Beth, who had received everyday injections in each of her shoulders for five years. Her medical medical doctor had never recommended another remedy, now not even PT! The kicker grow to be she responded so nicely to manual techniques that her sort of motion and ache had been superior with the aid of more than 50% in simplest one remedy. Beth's eyes nearly bugged out of her head as she felt her arm increase excessive without a pain inside the path of her preliminary consultation.

Steroid injections are not a fantastic concept for knee osteoarthritis, as years of steroid injections result in notably higher cartilage quantity loss and no huge distinction in knee pain in contrast with a saline placebo.forty

Medically manipulating infection with steroids does not deal with weak spot, imbalance, or each distinctive possible reason for the pain that you read about in Chapter 1. There are greater effective strategies to cope with this ache however without the risks, see Part three.

Spinal Cord Stimulators (SCS)

Spinal twine stimulator implants allow low-diploma electric currents to be done strategically, via wires, to the spinal twine.

The affected person then manages the currents the use of a much off manage. Theoretically, the currents disrupt ache signs from the body to the mind, which allows mask them.

A 2016 systematic examine of relevant literature published from 1966 thru March 2015 reviews most effective three studies were finished to assess the effectiveness of this system!41 One take a look at in comparison SCS to repeated lumbosacral spine surgical treatment for chronic ache.40 two The SCS commercial enterprise business enterprise changed into no better off whilst assessing each day lifestyles abilties and being able to artwork than the reoperation company, regardless of the truth that they confirmed tons less opioid use after surgical procedure. Isn't every day life function critical?

Another take a look at in comparison SCS mixed with traditional scientific control (CMM) to CMM by myself, and it determined that 32% of the SCS sufferers professional device-related complications.forty 3 CMM includes something that isn't surgical, along side ache drug treatments, chiropractic care, epidural injections, bodily therapy, and so on. The CMM treatment does now not specify the individual obtained capable physical remedy or amazing interventions that have been visible to be more effective.

The very last of the 3 research only compared high frequency (HF10) remedy to low frequency remedy, because of this that each groups underwent SCS strategies.40 four

Medical devices are a $four hundred billion business enterprise. About 34,000 patients go through SCS implants every twelve months global irrespective of they account for the 1/3-most variety of clinical tool damage reports to the U.S. Food and Drug Administration.45 Over 78,000 incidents have passed off given that 2008, together with shocks, burns, and spinal-twine nerve damage (beginning from muscle weakness to paraplegia). Hardware headaches are not unusual in almost forty% of sufferers, with the maximum common being unintentional movement of the leads. Other not unusual complications consist of failed connections or breakage of leads.46, 47

There is a way to block the mind's receipt of a ache message with out the need for surgical treatment. That is how TENS gadgets art work. A TENS (transcutaneous electric nerve stimulation) unit is a battery-powered device that clips in your belt, sits in your pocket, or is wrapped spherical a body thing. Typically, small electrodes that adhere to the pores and skin like band-aids are positioned strategically on the body. TENS can be very powerful at alleviating chronic ache with out the need for or the risks of surgical treatment.

Radiofrequency Ablation (RFA)

RFA is a way that destroys the nerve fibers wearing pain signals to the mind using warmth generated from alternating modern-day to ablate (get rid of) the tissue.

A assessment of 11 randomized, controlled trials checked out lower lower back pain, which includes disc ache, lumbar issue pain, and sacroiliac ache.forty eight-fifty two The cut price in pain rankings became no longer clear reduce in preference of RFA. When looking at disc pain,  out of 3 research confirmed no distinction. When searching at lumbar facet joint ache, most effective research showed development, and the others showed the manage institution did the equal or higher with out RFA. Studies for sacroiliac ache did not show promising outcomes both. One take a look at high-quality said a difference of 0.7 on a 0–10 scale. The distinctive have a look at said most effective   sufferers inside the treatment organization persisted to illustrate chronic pain consolation three hundred and sixty five days later. This is hardly ever a success story.

Risks of this treatment encompass harm to surrounding blood vessels and nerves, irreversible neurological harm that motives long-time period numbness and tingling, warm temperature damage to structures adjoining to the intention nerve, and muscular tissue harm.

I worked with a affected person, Cindy, for about 12 weeks, using on line conferences to remedy unrelenting neck and shoulder pain. She had a preceding nerve ablation method and although suffered intense pain that restricted her lifestyles and characteristic by means of the end of her workday, every day. Her weekends have been spent attempting to get over her operating week as an ultrasound technician. She had no remarkable of life till she discovered and professional in self-treatment strategies (shared in Part 3) over the direction of 15 training, which substantially transformed her worldwide.

Surgery

Common surgical techniques for pain are spinal fusions, arthroscopies, and laminectomies, but surgical treatment is often no longer powerful at reducing ache or restoring characteristic and may even add to the trouble.

Patients from thirteen clinics in eleven states with pain from herniated discs who did no longer have surgical remedy but had physical therapy, CBT counseling (cognitive behavioral remedy), and, in some times, took anti-inflammatory drugs. Forty percentage of these assigned to have surgical treatment did not have surgical operation due to the truth they advanced at the identical time as equipped.fifty 3 Other studies comparing spinal fusion surgical operation with rehabilitation determined no distinction in results.fifty four I suspect most human beings may choose workout over backbone surgical treatment any day.

What about knees? A test checked out humans with meniscal tears and in evaluation people who had surgical procedure vs. Folks that did now not.fifty 5 Patients had been randomized to get maintain of every arthroscopic partial meniscectomy (removal of torn shape) found with the resource of way of bodily therapy or a six-week physical remedy application best. The results have been about the equal for every companies. Again, which may also you choose, surgical remedy or no surgery?

According to a test published inside the New England Journal of Medicine, most of the 700,000 knee surgical techniques completed within the U.S. Each 12 months, at a charge of close to $four billion, are stated to be useless; no higher than sham surgical treatment.fifty six

All the ones joint replacements don't come with out dangers either. In the early 2000s, there was a don't forget of a metallic-on-steel hip opportunity implant especially designed for balance and longevity to treatment the project of hip replacements for younger/greater energetic people. This required additional surgical procedures to put off and replace this implant. Ouch!

Shockingly, joint alternative implants frequently come to marketplace with little to no clinical investigation. Most implant manufacturers use the 501(K) submission, additionally called the Premarket Notification (PMN), to pass the FDA's regulatory approval approach. As lengthy because of the truth the producer can usa that the modern tool is "appreciably identical" to modern gadgets on the market, they need no longer gift any medical statistics and the tool is permitted to marketplace. So a whole lot for affected character safety!

How approximately shoulders? In sufferers with isolated large posterior tears that are in the lower back of the shoulder (in desire to anterior tears inside the the the front), great benefits from rehabilitation remedy are stated.57 A shoulder decompression surgical treatment take a look at recommends at the least 3 to four months of nonsurgical treatment in advance than surgical operation, as patients who positioned tremendous attempt into nonsurgical remedies can also additionally keep away from surgical treatment.fifty 8

I sincerely have seen many human beings in immoderate ache get better without surgical treatment and resume entire functioning and ache-unfastened lives. This isn't to mention a person want to in no way have surgical treatment. The vital element is to be surely knowledgeable, efficiently cope with the foundation purpose (perpetrator), and ensure surgery is in truth critical to treatment the problem.

## Medical Imaging

Pain is frequently dealt with based totally totally on what is seen from imaging, that can affect diagnoses and effects. Let's see how beneficial X-rays, MRIs, and CT scans seem like. Spoiler alert! Medical imaging is regularly not consultant of the hassle. In specific terms, what's seen on imaging might not be the reason in your ache. For example, MRIs frequently find out small tears in knee meniscus, and tears are as not unusual in humans with out a pain as they're for humans with ache.fifty nine Also, arthritis is commonly answerable for hip pain, but most patients with not unusual hip pain do not show X-ray evidence of hip osteoarthritis (OA), and most patients with evidence of hip OA do no longer have common hip pain.60 Simply placed, X-ray effects and signs and symptoms do now not in shape.61 I actually have for my part treated many human beings with a diagnosis of arthritis and were able to alleviate their ache. I did no longer wave a magic wand over their OA.

Herniated discs are regularly blamed for returned ache while decided on imaging. A take a look at of MRIs for sufferers complaining of lower returned ache or leg ache refuted this. Some sufferers skilled pain after their herniated discs disappeared on imaging, while others said they felt higher, no matter the reality that the herniations had worsened.sixty   Hmmm. There turn out to be no relationship amongst pain and imaging consequences. Imagine having surgical remedy to your spine and the pain stays due to the truth the actual cause of your pain turned into never addressed?

Chronic low returned ache is often blamed on degenerative modifications, but X-rays, CT scans, and MRIs constantly show the presence of bulged/herniated discs, subluxations, scoliosis, osteoarthritis, pinched nerves, and so on, which all seem unrelated to whether or not or no longer a person stories continual ache.sixty three-sixty six

A 2013 have a look at on rotator cuff tears may also moreover wonder you; it bowled over me. The examine located that imaging determined out 147 topics had rotator cuff tears, however only fifty one of the 147 had signs and symptoms. The considered one of a type 96 people with rotator cuff tears had no signs and signs!67 In the overall population, 20% to forty% had rotator cuff tears without a signs and symptoms and signs.sixty eight,sixty nine This method shoulder pain may be efficaciously addressed without surgical treatment, due to the fact the symptoms may not be attributable to a tear.

Image

I desire this bankruptcy has been beneficial for you. While there are various pain remedy alternatives to pick from, plenty of them are much less than effective and may be downright risky. The accurate records is that there are techniques to deal with ache successfully, supplied in Part three, that do not include an extended listing of risky aspect effects.

It will pay to be informed. Your satisfactory path of movement is constantly to ask questions and then inform your healthcare company your preference that's based totally on being absolutely knowledgeable of all risks and blessings. Your provider does no longer need to certainly receive as real with you; exceptional to apprehend your preference. People are not used to speaking with their medical doctor in this manner, so in Resources, I endorse a video titled, "How to Have a Conversation with Your Doctor." You can also locate it quite helpful.

## Chapter 3: Treating Symptoms, Ignoring Causes, And Side Effects, Oh My!

Joan got here in to see me with a criticism of excessive leg pain. She emerge as depressing with an unrelenting, deep ache in each legs. It changed into affecting her sleep, her system, and her relationships. We did everything I must don't forget to solve her pain. I used more than one manual techniques similarly to modalities (at the side of warmth and ultrasound), but now not something positioned a dent inside the degree of pain she grow to be experiencing. Just once I changed into prepared to refer her to each different expert, she shared some component with me. She recommended me she had all started a present day remedy just in advance than the pain started out out. It have become a statin. She instructed her clinical medical doctor about the ache, stopped the drugs, and in three days her ache modified into long past! Joan grow to be ecstatic reporting this information to me. She had been given her existence once more!

If you take any over-the-counter or prescribed drugs for a continual situation that is identified to be better dealt with by way of way of food regimen and manner of life modifications, please recollect the subsequent facts. Millions of human beings turn out to be within the emergency room every 12 months after taking pharmaceuticals. In 2009, the National Institute on Drug Abuse stated near four.6 million drug-related ER visits, and nearly 50% were attributed to unfavorable reactions to medicinal tablets taken as prescribed.1

You may additionally additionally enjoy ache as a facet impact from taking a treatment for a medical condition, which then consequences in taking a ache treatment, which includes a danger of overdose and shortage of lifestyles ... and you could although have ache!

Even if the chance of overdose is not a difficulty, how about the side effect of persistent pain? I truly have had dozens of patients over time who've come to me because of moderate to excessive pain, and the reason was due to the aspect results of their treatment(s). I recollect it's vital to realise in case your modern-day drugs are inflicting your pain earlier than you looking for treatments on the way to be useless or, worse, dangerous.

Currently, 406 prescribed medicinal tablets list arthralgia (joint ache) as a side effect, and 253 listing again pain. There are many other painful thing outcomes, which incorporates myalgia (muscle ache), belly pain, testicular ache, spasms, and angina (chest pain). Many drugs additionally list the component consequences of weak point and fatigue, that may increase your threat of harm on the equal time as acting the smooth bodily responsibilities of every day lifestyles.

The following are currently usually prescribed drugs (with commonplace alternate names). The pinnacle 3 offered over 100 million prescriptions inside the U.S. In 2017 with the rest promoting between 40 and 80 million.

Lisinopril (Prinivil or Zestril)

- 

Atorvastatin (Lipitor) and Simvastatin (Zocor)

- 

Levothyroxine (Synthroid)

- 

Metformin (Glucophage)

- 

Amlodipine (Norvasc)

- 

Hydrochlorothiazide (HCTZ)

- Amoxicillin (Amoxil)

- Proton pump inhibitors (Nexium, Prevacid, Prilosec)

- Bisphosphonates (Actonel, Fosamax, Boniva, Reclast)

Medications for High Blood Pressure (Hypertension)

Lisinopril is prescribed to decrease blood pressure (BP) to lessen the threat of strokes and coronary coronary heart assaults; however, medically manipulating blood biomarkers (blood check consequences) does no longer lower your hazard as plenty as you will possibly count on. Improved biomarkers, and probable decreased stroke/cardiac sports, are decided but no huge difference in dying quotes.

What about the said ache element effects of this treatment?2 They consist of angina pectoris (chest ache), orthostatic hypotension (dizziness upon recognition with a chance of falls and damage), syncope (passing out), headache, and palpitations. Coughing is a commonplace purpose this treatment is discontinued and each other is prescribed to look if it's far higher tolerated.

The parameters for treating excessive BP keep to diagnose a symptom with out focusing at the motive. The cutting-edge parameters for prescribing treatment have real decrease BP readings as "disorder." Now that decrease BP readings are labeled "advanced," tens of thousands and thousands greater people may be prescribed antihypertensive drug treatments to manipulate their condition. I am not in competition to addressing the trouble; I am in the direction of in fact medicating the trouble and ignoring the remedy for the underlying purpose of the problem. Yes, I did write the phrase "remedy." When you have got high blood pressure, the endothelial cells that line your blood vessels are generating a lot less nitric oxide because of damage, which lets in your vessels to constrict, this is why your blood strain elevates. Rarely do I see absolutely everyone suggested to deal with this problem with nutritional changes (that are recognised to paintings), and as soon as the ones medicinal tablets are began, they hold for a lifetime. It is commonplace to preserve growing dosages and taken medicinal pills as BP readings hold to increase through the years.

Studies display endothelial sickness comes in advance than excessive blood stress, no longer the other way spherical.three Studies additionally display an accelerated consumption of plant-primarily based components and reduce of fatty food results in decrease BP.four Why isn't this in the headlines? I had a colleague who changed into on a medication for hypertension for 16 years. His wife took my Nourish magnificence, and the modifications she made of their own family meals enabled him to prevent taking the drugs, alongside collectively with his scientific medical doctor's blessing. His BP modified into now a healthful reading!

When it entails excessive blood stress and pain, folks who enjoy persistent pain have high blood pressure more frequently than those without continual pain.five In in any other case wholesome people (i.E., no particular chronic conditions as but identified), high blood pressure is visible to relate to having a diminished acute-ache threshold. This dwindled potential way you can sense ache extra extensively than a person without hypertension. (It's crucial to nation that if you have excessive blood stress however no unique acknowledged situations, you are not a healthy man or woman. There is underlying pathology occurring that may not have been seen or recognized.)

It isn't always sudden that the literature hyperlinks the superiority of ache in hypertensive individuals to medication factor results.6 Please recall, treating high blood pressure with capsules does not decrease your threat of lifestyles-changing fitness sports in a sizeable way. Addressing the underlying cause of the situation is essential in case your aim is to restore fitness and cast off the need for the medicine.

There are extraordinary unstable facet results that occur with those medicines. I'll use my patient Betty to demonstrate. I were running with Betty for severa weeks to deal with weak point problems. She had made awesome improvement going from looking to maintain onto something at some point of every workout to appearing over 30 minutes of sports fingers-loose. One day, she commenced her wearing activities as everyday. As I watched her perform actions she had completed effectively numerous instances earlier than, she started out to spin spherical heading inside the route of the ground. I turned into capable of draw near her and reduce her slowly to the floor just so she didn't get injured, thank God, however we have been each taken aback at what surely occurred. Then she knowledgeable me her medical doctor had changed her blood pressure medication days in advance and she or he have been dizzy ever considering the truth that. She in no way reported she changed into dizzy even as she arrived for our consultation. Her health practitioner emerge as in the same building, so wager wherein I located Betty to proper away? What if she had fallen within the automobile parking space or at domestic by myself and been injured? Not records the issue effects must have proved lethal.

Medications for Hyperlipidemia (High Cholesterol)

Atorvastatin and simvastatin are statins marketed to reduce "awful" cholesterol (LDL) and triglycerides, at the equal time as increasing levels of "pinnacle" ldl cholesterol (HDL) with the reason to lower your chance of stroke, coronary heart assault, and one of a kind coronary coronary heart complications. However, research display that decreasing ldl cholesterol with remedy will lessen your danger of a coronary heart attack, stroke, or loss of life thru much less than three%!7-10 You also can have advanced blood paintings even as your ranges are checked, however you are although at plenty the same chance you have been earlier than of experiencing a coronary coronary heart assault, stroke, or death. Medically manipulating blood biomarker ranges does not solve the motive you wanted the drug in the first area; however, a wholefood, plant-based totally eating regimen is robust at reducing your chance of experiencing an occasion or death.11,12

Let's check the ache aspect outcomes of statins. All statins have comparable results, however there are some variations cited inside the literature. For instance, Lipitor suggests cardiovascular and non-cardiovascular loss of existence as a usually pronounced factor effect (as a good deal as at the least one out of 10 experience this).thirteen Simvastatin, as an example, indicates angina (intense chest ache) as a commonplace thing impact.14,15

The most immoderate issue with statins is the musculoskeletal aspect results. They are myopathy (muscle illness resulting in weak spot), dermatomyositis (chronic muscle irritation and weak point), and rhabdomyolysis.16-18

Rhabdomyolysis, or the breakdown of muscle businesses, has signs of ache, weak spot, vomiting, confusion, kidney damage/failure, arthralgia (joint ache), myalgia (muscle ache), and tendon rupture (tendons be a part of muscle to bone). It is likewise probably lifestyles-threatening. Package inserts contain particular warnings about this hazard. But if the risks of occasions or dying are not decreased with the useful resource of any considerable quantity, is the medicine well worth it? This question ought to be requested throughout a intense dialogue along with your prescriber.

Other aspect effects of statins are belly ache,19-21 headache, peripheral neuropathy,22 chest pain, and testicular ache.23 You may need to know cognitive impairment, reminiscence loss,24-27 and impotence28 additionally arise.

If you have diabetes, you want to recognize that hyperglycemia is said in up to 10% of those taking atorvastatin (Lipitor). This manner an increase in your want for insulin and the consequent side consequences of that, that may be a higher threat of cardiac sports. I even have had patients with kind-2 diabetes who've been pretty upset once they located of this threat.

When looking on the numbers, there can be a 4% decrease in deaths and a 9% lower in a unmarried or extra essential coronary sports at the same time as evaluating simvastatin to placebo.29 The six-twelve months threat of survival changed into best 3.7% higher inside the statin agency. You should apprehend those statistics on the equal time as making decisions concerning your risks and benefits. If you experience that a 3.7% decrease danger is really worth it, then you without a doubt in the intervening time are making an knowledgeable choice.

I even have jumped via hoops often failing to help some sufferers with pain troubles, and ultimately, it grow to be placed their pain changed right right into a component impact from surely one among their medications. I now scrutinize all meds my affected person's listing on their assessment paperwork. If it's miles believed the medicinal drugs can be inflicting their ache, the subsequent step is to have a vital talk with their prescribing healthcare company to deal with the trouble thoroughly and accurately.

The most effective supply of ldl cholesterol in our weight loss plan is animal elements, because of this ingesting animal elements each day will increase your chance of developing excessive levels of cholesterol. Dr. John McDougall is a renowned health practitioner, author, and nutrients professional who has been reading, writing, and speakme approximately the results of nutrients on sickness for over 50 years. He informs readers on his internet site that they can anticipate to lower their ldl cholesterol diploma through the use of the use of 30 mg (if starting with a median of 220 mg) in fine two weeks with the aid of making the dietary modifications taught in his software program.30 If beginning with 240 mg or better, the not unusual decrease is forty mg. This information comes from analyzed bloodwork of 1700 folks who went thru the McDougall Residential Program in Santa Rosa, California.31

High ldl cholesterol will increase the chance of atherosclerosis, a unstable accumulation of ldl ldl ldl cholesterol and plaques on the walls of your arteries. Plaques reduce blood glide, impairing circulate to number one organs and everywhere and everywhere in your body. Impaired blood drift can result in life-converting headaches, along with coronary coronary heart attacks and strokes, further to loss of existence. Angina is a common symptom of atherosclerosis, which may be so intense that a person can enjoy unrelenting chest pain simply walking across a room. Talk approximately a lifestyles-proscribing painful state of affairs! There is likewise the issue of continual again ache due to impaired move to the lumbar arteries, that you first examine about in Chapter 1.

The essential fact to realize right here is that stepped forward ldl ldl cholesterol is a sign of horrible diet and impaired circulatory health. Lowering it with medicinal tablets does now not deal with the underlying motive of the difficulty or deal with pain in any practical way.

Medications for Hypothyroidism

Levothyroxine is given to deal with or prevent a goiter (enlarged thyroid gland), which can be as a result of hormone imbalances, radiation remedy, surgical treatment, or cancer.

According to the Mayo Clinic, hypothyroidism can make contributions to joint and muscle troubles.32 Hypothyroidism is stated to result in muscle aches, tenderness, and stiffness, in particular inside the shoulders and hips. It can also bring about joint pain and stiffness and swelling of the small joints inside the hands and ft. The most commonplace form of hypothyroidism, Hashimoto's thyroiditis, is an autoimmune (AI) hassle, and if a person has one AI problem, there can be a better incidence of developing unique AI troubles, in conjunction with rheumatoid arthritis.

According to the U.S. Preventive Services Task Force, there can be no dependable set of ordinary scientific signs and symptoms and symptoms that define thyroid sickness;33 regardless of the fact that, the threshold for diagnosis has been reduced, which has led to a full-size boom in the form of hypothyroid diagnoses.34 One take a look at anticipated that there are 1.6 million people inside the U.S. Who're currently medicated for hypothyroid disorder who do now not, in fact, have the disorder, and those people are much more likely to be harmed than helped thru remedy. So, in case you are in this medication, is it viable you can now not want it? A critical talk collectively with your prescriber can be so as.

Here are the ache (and a few terrific) trouble effects. Tachycardia (rapid coronary coronary heart rate), excessive blood strain, arrhythmia, coronary heart failure, angina (chest ache), myocardial infarction (coronary coronary heart assault), cardiac arrest (lack of lifestyles), complications, muscle prone point, muscle cramps, extended hazard of osteoporosis, and a immoderate fee of hip fractures.35-40

I certainly have  relative in her past due sixties with Hashimoto's, and she or he is pretty fitness conscious along side her diet and life-style. She works complete time and will be very busy with family. In spite of this health hassle, she has been capable of preserve herself quite wholesome and properly due to the fact she eats a wholefood, plant-based totally absolutely diet plan. This cute woman has a healthy weight, masses of strength, and takes first-rate thyroid medicinal drug.

Medications for Type-2 Diabetes

Metformin is prescribed in an attempt to beautify blood sugar manipulate in humans with kind-2 diabetes. It is every now and then utilized in mixture with insulin or particular medicines, but it is not for treating kind-1 diabetes, as it isn't insulin. This treatment does no longer resolve kind-2 diabetes and best lowers A1C stages through a median of one.Four.forty one A1C tests do not require fasting. They degree the amount of hemoglobin inside the blood that has glucose linked to it. One study suggests a beginning A1C diploma of eight.Eight have become decreased to 7.Four. A degree beneath five.7 is taken into consideration healthful, so losing a score from eight.Eight to 7.Four makes little fundamental fitness difference inside the scheme of things.

Getting the volume below five.7 wishes to be the goal.

Here are the pain (and a few different) element outcomes of Metformin. Lots of really commonplace digestive troubles, which incorporates diarrhea (fifty 3.2%), nausea/vomiting (25.Five%), and flatulence (12.1%). Common are indigestion, belly soreness, extraordinary stools, dyspepsia (belly pain), myalgia (muscle pain), chest discomfort, headache, and lightheadedness.42-47

The accurate facts is this situation is some thing you devour your manner into, because of this you can eat your manner out! I advise you look at Dr. Neal Barnard's Program for Reversing Diabetes, as this e-book offers the studies and specifics of what restores health. No medication that alters blood sugar ranges will repair your frame to health—however changing the manner you nourish your body can. Also via food plan, therefore, you may address the pain that incorporates diabetes.

Diabetic neuropathy is a common symptom of diabetes, affecting 60–70% of these with the ailment, in step with the National Institutes of Health.forty eight This ache can be devastating, as it's far steady, frequently intense, pain in arms or legs because of nerve damage with nerve function decline progressing over time. Tingling or numbness can stand up, in addition to pain inside the arms, palms, legs, or ft. Nerve harm also can arise in each organ device including your coronary coronary coronary heart, your digestive tract, even your sex organs. Peripheral neuropathy is the maximum commonplace form, and it will increase fall risk as a person won't be able to enjoy their toes on the floor. Not knowing in which your toes are in vicinity makes strolling and stability a actual assignment!

I am excited to percent a check that has shown extraordinary improvements on this very trouble the use of dietary intervention on my own.forty 9 This examine end up the primary randomized, managed test ever completed on the connection among food plan and diabetic nerve pain. (If you've got got were given or recognize a person who has diabetic nerve ache, you recognize how intense this pain may be and what form of it alters the excellent of lifestyles.) In this take a look at, the low-fat, plant-primarily based definitely weight loss plan business enterprise suggested a great improvement in pain: 80 one% on this employer said entire remission of burning ache and a sophisticated enjoy of touch (emphasis mine). The one of a kind 19% stated some improvement in symptoms. The development in signs modified proper into a 100% response charge!

Electrochemical pores and skin conductance (which checks one's potential to experience) in the foot worsened within the control business enterprise but stayed regular in the intervention group. This way the eating regimen may additionally additionally have slowed nerve function decline. This take a look at should be plastered inside the route of information headlines. Why isn't it?

There are forms of diabetes, type 1 and sort 2. Type 1 method your frame can not produce insulin, and you'll be depending on taking insulin for the relaxation of your lifestyles. Type 2 can imply you're "controlling" your scenario with eating regimen, taking oral medicinal tablets that have an effect on glucose levels, or taking insulin with the resource of injection. It all is based upon on your blood sugar ranges. Many studies display the effective impact of food plan on diabetes.50-fifty 5 Type 1 is also really induced thru weight loss program. You can lower the quantity of insulin required and decrease your hazard of all of the ones complications that coincide with the situation. Type-2 diabetics, who include 90% of all diabetics, can virtually do away with the symptoms and signs and symptoms in their scenario and remain nicely, with healthy dietweight-reduction plan.

Dr. Barnard's e-book gives countless studies displaying how beneficial the proper dietary conduct may be in addressing this circumstance. As you check only a 2d in the past, dietary intervention surely affects diabetic neuropathy quite effectively. If you be anxious with the aid of means of these issues, isn't it actually really worth seeing if this could be truly proper for you?

Neuropathy is not the nice "component impact" of diabetes. Other complications encompass a - to four-instances higher rate of dying from coronary coronary heart ailment/stroke, excessive blood stress, blindness because of diabetic retinopathy, kidney disorder and the want for dialysis, and amputation of limbs.

In my magnificence Nourish Your Body for Lifelong Wellbeing, I feed the beauty a four-path meal at the same time as they research the connection among food and ailment. I had a pupil in a single magnificence whose medical doctor desired to area him on Metformin because of the truth his A1C became better than ordinary. He counseled his medical medical doctor he desired to try converting his weight-reduction plan first, and he took my elegance because of the reality a coworker had encouraged it to him. After only some weeks, his A1C come to be everyday and his scientific medical doctor recommended him he come to be exceptional, no want for treatment. This guy had texted me several times from the grocery maintain with questions on what to buy: he took it considerably and it paid off. He even out of place thirty pounds!

Isn't it properly well well worth seeing if nutritional adjustments will be just right for you? See Resources.

Medication for Coronary Artery Disease

Amlodipine (e.G., Norvasc) dilates (widens) blood vessels and improves blood go along with the waft. It is used to deal with chest pain (angina) and exceptional situations due to coronary artery illness. Amlodipine is also used to deal with excessive blood pressure.

Side results of amlodipine encompass cardiovascular side outcomes, usually edema (swelling).56-fifty eight Swelling may be excruciating because of the stress on nerves. Other pain troubles are headache, peripheral neuropathy, belly ache, arthralgia (joint pain), myalgia (muscle ache), muscle cramps, and lower lower again pain.

For your data, even though now not a pain factor effect, impotence and sexual disorder are regularly seen with this drug.

Medication for Bacterial Infections

Amoxicillin, and different antibiotics, are used to deal with many special styles of infection as a consequence of micro organism, which consist of tonsillitis, bronchitis, pneumonia, gonorrhea, and infections of the ear, nostril, throat, skin, or urinary tract.

Antibiotics were a severe public-fitness issue for years. Many superbugs have passed off of past due which might be hard-to-address infections that don't respond nicely to antibiotics. Experts have relayed this case about the over-prescribing of these tablets. If you have got a lifestyles-threatening contamination, antibiotics can preserve your life. If you have got were given a mild contamination research have verified will remedy on its personal, antibiotics might not be a worthwhile opportunity due to the damaging effects for your immune tool and digestive tract. There is likewise the superiority of antibiotic use in the animals we devour, due to this you are ingesting antibiotics every day if you devour a trendy American food plan.

Pain factor consequences of antibiotics are stomach pain, vulvovaginal mycotic contamination (yeast contamination, which can be very painful), headache, and joint pain.59,60

Medications for Edema (Swelling)

HCTZ (hydrochlorothiazide) lets in save you your frame from absorbing too much salt, that could result in fluid retention. It is prescribed for congestive coronary coronary heart failure, cirrhosis of the liver, kidney disorders, edema due to the element effects of taking steroids or estrogen, and excessive blood pressure.

There are plenty of extensive side results with this drug.61-sixty seven If you've got were given troubles collectively along side your levels of cholesterol, be warned that this drug is thought to increase ordinary serum cholesterol via 11%, LDL lipoprotein ldl ldl cholesterol by way of 12%, and VLDL lipoprotein levels of cholesterol thru 50%. If you have got diabetes, you want to recognize it could reduce insulin secretion, and real glucose intolerance may additionally growth in approximately 3% of patients. It is typically reversible internal six months after discontinuation of treatment, however six months is a long term to remedy a medicinal drug facet impact, don't you think?

Scarily, this drug has a mortality rate of 6%, and some experts say this is grossly underreported.

While death is the most important trouble there are a couple of ache aspect outcomes to mention at the side of muscle spasm and myalgia (muscle ache).68,69 There are also issues with weak point, vertigo, paresthesia, dizziness, headache, cognitive impairment, and bone mineral density.70-seventy four

Medications for Bone Density

On January 7, 2008, the us Food and Drug Administration alerted healthcare specialists and clients to the uncommon immoderate element outcomes of a famous elegance of medicine for osteoporosis and Paget's sickness: the bisphosphonate (Actonel, Fosamax, Boniva, Reclast). They can purpose "severe and occasionally incapacitating bone, joint, and muscle pain," which "may also arise inner days, months, or years" after first taking the medicine.

This medication has nearly truly described a few in any other case inexplicable pain in a number of my patients through the years. Alendronate and risedronate (Actonel) are the two most well-known bisphosphonates. If you're over 40 and grappling with a brilliant ache trouble, check your treatment cabinet for bisphosphonates.

My mother end up prescribed this kind of capsules, and he or she or he ended up within the ER due to the fact she concept she emerge as having a coronary heart assault from the chest ache component impact. The drug had broken her esophagus. You can consider how this terrified her, as my brother died from most cancers and the number one internet internet site on line grow to be his esophagus.

Other jaw-losing (no pun meant) side consequences of these capsules are osteonecrosis of the jaw (bone lack of lifestyles) and unusual thigh bone fractures, to name simply .

Low bone density isn't what you can had been precipitated trust. If you would love to observe greater visit Resources for records about a free PDF.

Medications for Reflux

Gastroesophageal reflux disease (GERD) is pretty often a issue effect of drug treatments prescribed for distinct conditions.seventy five-seventy nine The maximum common are antibiotics, NSAIDs (anti inflammatory ache relievers), bisphosphonates (osteoporosis meds), potassium chloride, and iron supplements because of the reality the ones medicinal pills are caustic.

Pill-brought approximately reflux is not the handiest reason reflux occurs. There are other reasons, which includes extended pressure on your lower esophageal sphincter (LES), which motives it to open while it shouldn't. This effects in belly acid contacting your esophagus. What places pressure to your sphincter? Excess belly fats, pregnancy, constipation, and overfilling your belly at some stage in meals. Liquids ate up with meals can be a part of the overfilling. Medications intention to growth the charge of emptying acids from the belly or inhibit/block stomach acid manufacturing. Unfortunately, this makes it greater difficult in your body to digest food properly as acid is needed for proper digestion.

## Chapter 4: The Physiology Of Pain

The handiest definition of ache is a few element that hurts. The word is thought to originate from the Latin poena or the Greek poine, which each take a look at with pain from punishment or penalty. Pain is synonymous with damage, pain, and any unsightly sensation. More severe tiers of ache are related to terms which incorporates "distress" and "suffering."

As there are numerous tiers of pain, from moderate to agonizing, there too are various developments of ache. It can be dull, sharp, throbbing, smarting, pinching, stabbing, taking pictures, cramping, and so forth. Pain that is everyday and constant is commonly known as an pain.

We all understand what pain is, due to the fact every person have professional it. The more exciting query is, Where does ache come from? According to scientists, pain is the stop end end result of the stimulation of precise receptors in our frame. There are limitless receptors in our body which is probably touchy to positive stimuli. Some receptors sense temperature, others experience pressure, and despite the fact that others revel in ache. Many of those receptors are discovered at the skin floor. They are activated at the same time as adjustments in stress, temperature and unique variables are felt thru some a part of our frame. For example, pain receptors are stimulated whilst a heavy strain bears down on our lap, or whilst we step on a few trouble sharp or hot. These receptors are also set off whilst sure chemical substances are released with the useful resource of manner of injured cells in our frame.

When inspired, pain receptors supply a sign that travels alongside our spinal cord until it reaches our thoughts. Upon reaching the mind, the sign is interpreted as pain, and the mind then problems a corresponding reaction. This reaction is often a command to move some distance from the object that reasons the ache.

Let's look at an instance. When your finger touches a sharp item, this stimulates ache receptors positioned in your finger. The ache receptors ship a join up your mind thru nerve pathways along your spinal cord. In reaction, the mind problems a command to the muscle corporations in your finger to withdraw from the needle.

The loop along which the indicators (or nerve impulses) excursion is referred to as the "ache pathway." These signals tour right away, in milliseconds, such that it every so often takes a second for us to experience the pain of a pinprick and then react through moving an extended way from the item inflicting it.

An thrilling minutiae is that the mind itself does not have ache receptors. Thus, poking at the brain (if this had been viable) could not cause the ache mechanism described above.

The technical time period for peripheral pain receptors, regarding the ones which can be determined on or close to the pores and pores and skin ground, is nociceptors. As stated, they will be very touchy to outside stimuli which include modifications in temperature or stress. The ache they bring about is known as nociceptive ache. There is every other form of pain, referred to as non-nociceptive, that isn't right away related to the stimulation of peripheral receptors. Non-nociceptive pain is generally because of an harm or damage interior our frame. Some of the subjects which can cause this pain are sprains, muscle cramps, bone breakage, nerve harm, tissue infection, organ disease, and lack of oxygen.

You might also have heard of our frame's herbal inflammatory response. This is stimulated whenever there may be damage, trauma or contamination in any a part of the frame. It is a natural mechanism presupposed to deal with the harm and repair the injured body component returned to a healthful nation. As a part of the inflammatory response, our body releases hormones referred to as prostaglandins. Unfortunately, while prostaglandins are at artwork, they reason pain further to swelling, fever and distinct symptoms and signs of infection. Prostaglandins also heighten the sensitivity of pain receptors.

Some ache relievers artwork by way of way of way of suppressing the movement of prostaglandins. These drugs lessen or do away with ache, similarly to the fever and swelling that often accompany it. Examples of these analgesics (the scientific term for painkillers) are paracetamol and ibuprofen.

In a comparable fashion, other ache relievers art work via numbing ache receptors on our pores and pores and skin or on a localized a part of our body. Anesthetics are an example of this kind of remedy. Their impact is short; after a while, the ache receptors come to be energetic all over again, and the person can feel ache and one in every of a type sensations in that part of his frame once more.

We see proper proper here that ache can be relieved or averted while the pain pathway is obstructed in some manner. When the pain receptors are desensitized, they can not send "pain messages" to the mind. When the discharge of prostaglandins is averted, they can not cause ache.

All this is right, but we have to also recognize that ache serves an outstanding cause. For one issue, it certainly works to warn the us capability chance. If you located your hand on a warm range and also you don't sense any pain, you received't apprehend that this is risky and you can get a nasty burn (or possibly lose your hand!). If we habitually suppress our frame's inflammatory reaction (which encompass prostaglandins), we inhibit the herbal recovery method. Thus, we need to be cautious in treating ache, mainly at the same time as unsupervised via a systematic practitioner.

Types of Pain

Not all types of ache are identical. If we're lucky, we get the slight and brief-lived kinds. Some humans have debilitating continual ache that they have to go through for so long as they stay.

The only training of pain are acute and persistent. Acute pain is brief-lived, however has a bent to be extra immoderate. Most acute pain accompanies an harm. When the harm is healed, the pain goes away, too. Chronic pain lasts for lots longer durations. It can disappear, and then recur, time and again. It is typically an entire lot less immoderate than acute pain, irrespective of the fact that a few kinds of chronic ache may be very immoderate as well.

In the primary bankruptcy, we talked of nociceptors. These receptors cause nociceptive pain, of which there are essential types: somatic and visceral.

Somatic pain refers to pain felt at the pores and skin or the musculo-skeletal device. This pain is due to immoderate warm temperature or cold, pressure, and stretch in the muscle groups. Skin cuts, muscle tears and tissue damage can also purpose somatic pain. Muscle cramps, which is probably regularly skilled thru the use of athletes, are each extraordinary example of somatic pain. The purpose of cramps is often oxygen depletion in the affected muscle corporations. Most kinds of somatic pain are acutely painful. Thankfully, they're normally localized to a small a part of the frame. When this element is touched or moved, the ache generally will growth.

Meanwhile, visceral pain originates from someplace deeper inside the body, together with the inner organs, the belly, the thorax and the pelvic vicinity. Compared to somatic ache, visceral pain isn't as localized, and it has a bent to be more an pain than a pointy shape of ache. Some examples of visceral pain are colic, menstrual cramps, and returned ache.

Moving on to non-nociceptive pain, or ache that isn't attributable to the motion of nociceptors, we have were given nerve or neuropathic ache. This pain originates from the involved tool. Examples are pain due to worried problems or conditions, which incorporates a couple of sclerosis, a slipped disc within the spinal column, shingles, and stroke. Nerve ache is complicated because of the involvement of the frightened machine, the very mechanism in rate of the transmission of ache alerts. When this device turns into compromised in a few manner, the signaling mechanism furthermore will become unstable and messed up. This can also purpose specific symptoms and symptoms, consisting of numbness, tingling sensations, pins and needles, and diverse hypersensitivities. These symptoms and signs and symptoms, as well as the ache, have a propensity to arise haphazardly.

Another form of non-nociceptive pain is sympathetic pain. This includes each different a part of the nervous tool that is referred to as the sympathetic worrying gadget. Here, sure nerves are malfunctioning, resulting inside the random, unstable firing off of impulses to the thoughts, which might be interpreted as ache. This can be very excessive, due to the truth sympathetic nerves control the functioning of our pores and skin and

muscle organizations. Damage to the ones nerves need to result in the immobility of the affected limbs. This type of ache is related to sicknesses which consist of osteoporosis and arthritis.

Yet a few extraordinary shape of pain is referred or reflective pain. This is ache felt not on the injured or diseased body element, however near it. For example, a person who has harm his shoulder may additionally moreover enjoy the ache not at the shoulder however in his arm or inside the neck region. Similarly, someone having a coronary heart attack might not sense pain in his chest, however alternatively on his neck or shoulders. Interesting, as much as this time, scientists have now not however understood why referred pain happens.

Meanwhile, radiating pain is one that is felt every on the inspiration of the trauma or contamination and within the surrounding regions. This too can arise within the direction of a coronary heart assault, even as the man or woman feels pain in the chest, the shoulders, the decrease again and the neck. Because a bigger region of the body is concerned, radiating pain can be pretty distressing.

Finally, a few scientific doctors use the terms "fast ache" and "slow ache." Without getting too technical, speedy pain is acute and frequently involves the pores and skin and mouth, and is due to the motion of pain receptors. Skin tears, as an instance, can motive speedy ache. Once the tear is healed, the ache is long gone. On the opposite hand, sluggish pain is generally felt within the internal organs, and is non-nociceptive. This pain may also be felt as referred or radiating. A ideal instance is the ache felt with the aid of moms-to-be at some point of exertions.

## Chapter 5: Common Pharmacological Treatments For Pain

The remedy given for ache relies upon on many things. The doctor asks the individual to offer an reason behind the pain, in which it's miles felt, how prolonged it is been there, and if there's a suspected reason that would provide an reason behind it. Because pain is subjective, the medical doctor listens cautiously to how his affected person describes it. Pain is what the patients says it's miles, regardless of what the physician or any other character might also moreover agree with.

Rating scales are used to assist patients precise the amount of ache they feel. The maximum common among those are numerical score scales of zero to ten. A 0 way no pain, five approach slight pain, and ten method the most excessive ache potential. For children, faces scale are greater appropriate. They are established faces with expressions frequently beginning from glad (no pain) to agonized (immoderate pain). They then are informed to pick which face corresponds to how they revel in.

Afterwards, the medical doctor examines the patient and takes into attention one-of-a-kind signs and signs and symptoms that can be gift. If crucial, laboratory tests are completed. In most instances, the physician is then capable of become privy to the person and reason of the ache and prescribe the ideal ache reliever.

If the pain is due to an underlying disorder, pain relievers aren't the handiest prescription given with the aid of the medical doctor. Treatment for the sickness should also be supplied, and this normally receives rid of the ache in due time.

The not unusual medicinal capsules for pain are listed under. Many of these are to be had over-the-counter, at the same time as a few need to be prescribed by way of the usage of a medical doctor.

Non-opioid Analgesics

These provide relief for nociceptive ache, however no longer for nerve ache. Thus, they're generally used for not unusual pains professional through maximum people, at the side of headaches, muscle pains, cramps and fever.

They deal with moderate to slight pain.

They are non-addictive. As such, they may be regular to apply as long as the individual adheres to the endorsed dosage.

Common examples are Tylenol (acetaminophen), non-steroidal anti-inflammatory tablets or NSAIDs (ibuprofen), COX-2 inhibitors, and salicylates (aspirin). Most of these are available over the counter without the need for a medical doctor's prescription.

While NSAIDs are significantly used, they're able to have element outcomes that embody gastro-intestinal bleeding and stomach issues. COX-2 inhibitors have a decrease danger of gastro-intestinal component outcomes. The use of salicylates can result in certain thing consequences which embody kidney and gastro-intestinal troubles. But in low doses, the ones drug treatments are usually stable.

High doses of these capsules require a doctor's prescription. Older sufferers want to in particular be monitored carefully at the same time as taking excessive doses due to the truth they may be extra vulnerable to the unsightly aspect results.

Opioid Analgesics

Also referred to as opiates, those are narcotics supposed to remedy severe pain. Examples are morphine, oxycodone and methadone.

They are very robust painkillers that need to be administered best via licensed scientific practitioners. They are normally utilized in surgical tactics, cancer treatment (chemotherapy), bone remedy, and for burn patients.

Small doses are administered first. They are progressively progressed until ache remedy is completed. In ultra-cutting-edge, nice very low doses are given to babies and the aged.

The everyday aspect consequences of opioids are drowsiness, nausea, itching, constipation, and the risk of developing a dependence at the drug. The patient can show withdrawal signs and symptoms if manage of the drug is unexpectedly stopped. As such, a tapering-off duration is regularly located.

When the severity of the pain decreases, the clinical doctor replaces the ache medicinal drug with a non-opioid analgesic.

Anti-epileptic, anti-tension and anti-depressant drug remedies

Some capsules used to address epilepsy, anxiety and melancholy also are used to deal with continual and neuropathic pain.

Examples are gabapentin (an anti-epileptic), Valium (an anti-anxiety), and trazodone (an anti-depressant).

This treatment want to be carefully monitored by way of manner of a health practitioner. There are more feasible issue effects, and a taper-off length is in truth important to prevent seizures.

Other analgesics

Studies have validated that medical marijuana (a cannabinoid) is an powerful treatment for chronic pain.

Some muscle relaxants collectively with orphenadrine and cyclobenzaprine are beneficial in treating musculo-skeletal pain.

These pills can be used collectively with an opioid, beneath near scientific supervision. They are regarded to "potentiate" or boom the effectiveness of opioids.

## Chapter 6: Alternative Treatments For Pain

Non-pharmacological ache treatment is an opportunity for people who do not like to take drugs, or who can not do so because of scientific reasons. People with kidney and liver troubles, as an example, are usually recommended to keep away from high-quality analgesics because of the truth the usage of the ones can aggravate their pre-current scientific scenario.

In awesome cases, opportunity treatments can be used together with analgesic drugs. This -pronged technique quickens ache consolation.

Below are some non-drug remedy alternatives for the control of pain.

Electricity – Studies have proven that the use of strength to stimulate positive mind areas outcomes within the release of herbal materials that act like opioids. This therapy is strong for migraines and pains within the face or head location. Transcutaneous electric nerve stimulation (TENS) is a model of this treatment. Here, low-voltage current is completed on the pores and skin near the deliver of ache. TENS is in particular effective for the relaxation of pain related to diabetic neuropathy.

Acupuncture – Based on age-antique Chinese traditional remedy, acupuncture works through placing needles into precise factors at the pores and skin. There is sufficient anecdotal evidence to resource its effectiveness, however the way it really works and why haven't begun to be understood via current scientists.

Exercise – This facilitates to lessen pain through growing flexibility and muscle electricity. It additionally works thru freeing hormones referred to as endorphins. These "glad hormones" are natural painkillers.

Cognitive behavioral treatment (CBT) – This is a shape of therapy in which the affected person spends time with a psychiatrist in seeking to understand the relationship of the pain he's experiencing and his thoughts, emotions and moves. Alternative techniques of thinking, way of lifestyles changes, rest techniques, and new coping techniques are superior to help the person manipulate his pain and specific fitness troubles.

Physical treatment— This involves techniques to enhance physical feature or moves weakened thru an harm.

Hypnosis — Still a arguable pain treatment, hypnosis has despite the fact that been shown to be powerful in clinical trials. Patients that blanketed kids and teenagers with continual pain skilled dramatically decreased pain after hypnosis.

Visualization and relaxation strategies — These assist to lower pain as the thoughts makes a speciality of harmonious, exciting images. They are beneficial within the remedy of persistent ache. Meditation and yoga are well-known examples of those ache control strategies.

Massage – This is every other rest method that may soothe or stimulate worn-out muscle agencies to decrease pain. There are numerous styles of rubdown, collectively with difficult and moderate kinds, deep tissue, Thai, Swedish and shiatsu.

Chiropractic remedy – This might be very powerful in particular for decrease back pain. Chiropractors are certified practitioners who manipulate the frame to repair the most efficient alignment of bones and tissues.

Reiki recovery – This is an strength-primarily based completely opportunity treatment that promotes natural self-recuperation. It is perception to now not terrific relieve ache but additionally remedy chronic ailments and restore vigour.

Natural and Home Treatments for Pain

For slight to moderate pain, most people depend upon over-the-counter tablets. These are easy to get, specially stable, and powerful if used well. For excessive pain, the right element to do is to seek advice from a clinical doctor and feature him devise the best treatment plan. This plan need to flip out to consist of the usage of analgesic drugs, or a non-pharmacological approach, or a combination of the two. It may also incorporate more unconventional ache treatment plans, specially in the case of continual pain that does not appear like relieved with general ache remedies.

As an accent to the traditional techniques of relieving pain, everyone can also attempt out some natural treatments that can be finished at domestic using clean materials. While some of those substances won't be pretty clearly determined in a single's treatment cabinet or kitchen, they may be without problem procured in herbal shops or pharmacies.

Below are a few stable and herbal pointers that might help relieve pain:

Take glucosamine sulfate and chondroitin sulfate nutritional dietary supplements. These herbal compounds are regarded to ease knee and joint pain associated with arthritis. At the same time, they increase joint mobility. There are not any said terrible outcomes from taking the ones dietary dietary supplements.

Also hold in mind taking fish oil dietary dietary supplements. This have useful fatty acids and anti inflammatory sellers that assist to lubricate the joints and ease pain.

A vegetarian diet is beneficial in relieving menstrual cramps and pain related to high-quality illnesses collectively with fibromyalgia and osteoarthritis.

Take herbs together with turmeric, ginger and black pepper. You can add those to the meals which you commonly consume. Like fish oil, those herbs have anti inflammatory houses that help to lessen ache.

Eat more pink grapes, blueberries and cranberries. These have a compound known as resveratrol, this is especially beneficial to human beings stricken by spinal disc problems. Resveratrol additionally permits in tissue restore.

Indulge in goodies occasionally, but don't make a addiction of it. For a few reason, consuming cookies, chocolate and ice cream has been located to lessen someone's perception of pain. Even just the odor of home-baked cookies can assist to decrease ache.

Take day out for normal massages. This smooth pain comfort method permits to relieve all types of pain, together with tension complications, again pain, neck ache, and muscle ache related to sports activities activities sports and exercise. Because massages are very relaxing, additionally they assist promote a great night time time's sleep, which similarly facilitates restore the body to health.

Also make the effort to do normal exercising. Like massage, exercising releases endorphins and serotonin. These are hormones that now not only make us revel in extraordinary however additionally relieve ache truly. They are chargeable for the herbal excessive that runners enjoy after an active workout. Moreover, they assist ease anxiety and depression. Some endorsed exercising sports are walking, walking, tai chi and qigong. Choose one which isn't always too strenuous for you.

Engage in yoga or meditation. These are very exciting sports activities that assist to ease pain and decrease pressure degrees. Yoga is in particular suitable for lower back ache and headaches. Meanwhile, meditative techniques that alter respiration and calm the thoughts produce many advantages for our health and well being.

Meditation lets in someone manipulate ache with the aid of focusing his interest faraway from the ache and on something unbiased or greater remarkable. It is fantastic for continual pain patients.

Spend time with pals, or make new ones. Social touch has been examined to help people with persistent ache. If the humans you keep out with have the same contamination or revel in comparable symptoms and signs that you have, then this shared contact is all of the more together beneficial. Online organizations and dialogue forums are an incredible venue to get to apprehend different human beings with the identical health troubles.

Use warm temperature remedy. Pour hot water in a bottle, or get a gel-filled pad and heat it inside the microwave, and then region it in opposition to any part of your body that feels painful. The heat will growth blood go along with the go with the flow and oxygen supply to that part of your frame, which then eases any pain and makes the ache leave quicker. Instead of using a water bottle or a pad, you may in reality take a warm tub. Heat treatment must be accomplished not than 20 mins.

Use bloodless remedy. Alternatively, you can comply with ice or cold compress on any painful part of your frame. This relieves inflammation and pain. It additionally reduces pain through slowing down the transmission of nerve impulses. Again, do now not use cold remedy for extra than 15 to twenty mins at a time. Around ten minutes need to suffice. If favored, you could repeat the method after resting for approximately 15 minutes.

Take Vitamin D supplements and go outdoors. Sunlight is critical for the absorption of Vitamin D and calcium, which can be vitamins important for bone health. Women with osteoarthritis and comparable bone situations need to spend a while outside and take the multivitamin supplementation appropriate for his or her age. A minimal of about 15 minutes under the sun is commonly recommended every day.

Make tremendous that you get seven to 9 hours of sleep every night. The type of hours of sleep each one people dreams varies, however it typically isn't lower than seven hours. Sleep is restorative and healing. If you discover it tough to get an high-quality night time time's sleep, bear in thoughts taking on rest sports like meditation and yoga. Exercise additionally helps to sell top sleep.

Learn ache control strategies via highbrow imagery and visualization. An instance is changing your awareness. This without a doubt consists of focusing on part of your frame this is pain-free. If you've got once more ache, cognizance on your ft (or some specific body element). In your mind, you could do whatever on the facet of your feet to preserve your attention far from your once more ache. You can take delivery of as true together with your ft being suffused with warm temperature, or turning blue. Feel loose to allow your creativeness and visualization run wild. Another technique is to depend backwards from a hundred, or to recite the alphabet backwards. The concept is to interact your mind far from the ache. You also can mentally recite nursery rhymes, do arithmetic, make a to-do listing, and so on. You can get as revolutionary or as mundane as you please, good-bye as it takes continues your thoughts

## Chapter 7: The History Of Marijuana

Cannabis sativa is the clinical name of the hemp plant. There are extraordinary forms of hemp plants but cannabis is the maximum normally used one. Just from its call, sativa technique useful and hashish method hemp. It grows within the wild in tropical and temperate areas.

Hemp is any durable plant that has been in existence for the motive that ancient instances. It's most famous byproduct is fiber, and ropes are made from the hemp plant.

The hashish is the most long lasting form of hemp. It produces the canvas, taken into consideration to be the hardest cloth, that is commonly used to make sails. Cannabis pulp is applied as gasoline and is an crucial issue in making paper. The seed is used for meals. The oil extracted from the seed can be used for paints and varnishes. Cannabis moreover has medicinal residences.

The Many Uses of Cannabis

As meals

The seed is an superb deliver of protein. The seeds are eaten via oatmeal. It is with out problems digestible and doesn't provide you with the "excessive" that you could get from smoking dried leaves. Cannabis seed is likewise a great deliver of essential fatty acids. It is used as meals dietary supplements. Regular intake reduces the threat of developing coronary heart troubles. Cannabis doesn't need fertilizer to expand, consequently, it charges less in comparison to one of a kind vegetables that want greater renovation.

As cloth

The stalk of the cannabis plant is an notable source of fabric. It includes additives, the bast and the hurd (pulp). Bast or fiber is woven to make a completely long lasting sort of material. Did you understand that the primary Levi's denims were made from hashish bast?

Useful element to make paper

The cannabis fiber and pulp are used to make paper. The first paper made from hashish changed into created in historical China. Paper made from fiber can be very long lasting, despite the fact that thin and brittle. Paper made from pulp isn't always as robust as the only made from fiber but it's far a good deal less complex to make. Pulp paper is softer and thicker and is used for lots of tremendous purposes. The modern-day-day day paper which you use these days is made from chemical pulp from wooden.

As gasoline

Cannabis pulp may be used to make gas. It is burned as is or it's far processed to create charcoal, methane gasoline, methanol, and gas. It undergoes a manner of damaging distillation to manufacture fuel.

As treatment

Marijuana became legally used till 1937 because of the medicinal residences that it consists of. It became presented as nerve tonic decrease again then. It modified into considered to be an splendid treatment for quite some illnesses, which include sclerosis, glaucoma, epilepsy, allergic reactions, migraine headaches, dystonia, and ache. The maximum commonplace medicinal software program is to relieve vomiting and nausea. Extraction modified into particularly clean and the extracts can be used as thing to make food, drinks, butter, or even alcohol. It moreover has very powerful disinfecting houses.

## Chapter 8: Marijuana Basics

What is marijuana?

The dried flowers and leaves of hashish sativa are referred to as marijuana. It is normally smoked in hand-rolled cigarettes, generally known as joints. It is also called grass, dope, pot, weed, Mary Jane, smoke, green, joints, and heads.

A lot of human beings smoke marijuana to provide them a sense of euphoric experience or a unique form of "immoderate". Some say, smoking marijuana allows them to loosen up. Cannabis alters the customers notion and causes rest. Smoking pot also can bring about paranoia and hallucinations.

Marijuana is the most commonplace unlawful substance inside the United States. Studies display that at the least a 3rd of the American population has smoked marijuana eventually of their lives.

What are the effects of smoking marijuana?

Potential brief-term results:

•Anxiety

•Paranoia

- Memory impairment

- Learning difficulties

- Lack of awareness and attention

- Poor the usage of abilties

- Poor motor talents

- Difficulty concentrating

- Drowsiness

- Loss of coordination

- Bloodshot (red) eyes

- Dryness of the mouth and throat

- Increase in urge for food

- Decreased nausea

## Chapter 9: Medicinal Marijuana And Pain Management

Twenty of the 50 US states have legalized the use of marijuana for medicinal abilities for the motive that 1972. Those who useful resource the use of marijuana for its medicinal homes argue that this most well-known hemp plant is a stable and really powerful remedy for a couple of sclerosis, AIDS, glaucoma, a few forms of most cancers, and persistent ache. Their arguments are backed by using big researches and studies.

The use of opportunity remedy dates returned to historic instances at the same time as Chinese treatment become introduced. Today, opportunity remedy remains very famous to relieve tremendous illnesses. Aromatherapy and acupuncture are of the most famous opportunity picks. The use of medicinal herbs stays popular in todays society

Cannabis has been used and taken into consideration to be a "magical herb" because of its numerous medicinal uses. Though its use remains unlawful in some states, its clamor to be used because of its medicinal houses continues till nowadays.

Here are in reality 5 of the maximum commonplace ailments that medicinal marijuana can be very effective in treating:

1.Vomiting and Nausea

Your frame has  types of receptors, CB1 and CB2 receptors. These receptors permit your frame to take in the consequences of cannabis. CB1 receptors are determined on your thoughts and your spinal wire, on the equal time as CB2 receptors are to your immune tool. As the body comes in contact with the marijuana, your frame will produce endocannabinoids, the molecules that allows you to interact along side your CB1 and CB2 receptors. You may be delivered proper right into a euphoric nation if you want to block off the symptoms and symptoms and signs and symptoms of nausea and vomiting. This remedy is normally endorsed to maximum cancers patients present process chemotherapy to ease chemo-related-vomiting and nausea. It is said to be extra effective than maximum of the FDA standard anti-nausea drugs available within the mainstream marketplace these days.

1.Appetite stimulant

There are studies achieved in HIV excessive quality and AIDS patients who've had immoderate weight loss that display an growth in their urge for food on the same time as given dietary dietary supplements with medicinal cannabis. It has additionally been effective in most cancers sufferers. There is also proof that the inhalation of marijuana consequences in improved calorie-consumption.

1.Spasm and muscle anxiety remedy

Another medicinal software program of marijuana is to offer remedy from muscle anxiety and spasm. Patients who've multiple sclerosis had been said to have skilled a marked decrease in shaking and muscle spasms upon consumption of the liquid extract with THC and cannabidiol. Medicinal marijuana has additionally been determined to lower muscle stiffness and tremors.

1.Chronic ache

Cannabis has extended been believed to be an effective analgesic that alleviates persistent pain. People who complain of neuropathic pain, generally because of backbone surgery, amputation, and alcoholism, have located treatment from the use of medicinal marijuana.

1.Treatment for insomnia

People smoke marijuana because of its relaxation results. Medicinal marijuana has moreover been discovered to help relieve symptoms and signs and symptoms and signs of depression and tension and insomnia. Studies display that the ones folks who "smoked" marijuana showed marked enhancements in their moods had been capable of get a better sleep.

Medicinal marijuana has additionally been powerful in treating the following:

•Anorexia

•Arthritis

•Alzheimer's disease

•Crohn's disease

•Migraine

•Fibromyalgia

Should marijuana be taken into consideration for its medicinal benefits?

Despite its addictive risks, proponents of medicinal marijuana maintain to push for its entire legalization to deal with illnesses. What pretty some people do no longer admire is that marijuana has remarkable healing substances which may be useful to man.

Back in the 70's, a synthetic version of THC, it certainly is the principle substance in hashish that gives its medicinal houses, became synthesized to be used as drug known as Marinol. However, due to the truth the usage of marijuana is illegal, the drugs, for a time, emerge as likewise limited from the general market. Today, more and more states are recognizing the fine effects of medicinal marijuana. Proponents had been pushing its production, cultivation, and use for medicinal functions.

Proponents of medicinal marijuana preserve to push for research with the intention to dispute the perception that marijuana is addictive.. In fact, there are studies already that display using cannabis as an powerful remedy for heroin addiction.

Marijuana may be used for neurological situations, like epilepsy due to its anticonvulsant homes. There are also brand new studies that show its benefits in assuaging premenstrual syndrome and excessive blood pressure.

As said earlier, there are 20 US states that lets in the use of medicinal marijuana. More and further human beings are seeing the health and clinical benefits of the hashish plant.

One of the number one reasons for its increasing recognition is its powerful use for ache manipulate. Pain can come from a number of one-of-a-kind clinical situations, like complications, maximum cancers, nerve pain, and glaucoma.

Doctors suggest the usage of medicinal marijuana for the remedy of the subsequent:

•Muscle spasms because of multiple sclerosis

•Nausea and vomiting after a chemotherapy session

•Extreme weight reduction due to a continual infection and nerve pain

•Seizures

It is vital to be aware that the FDA gave its approval for the usage of THC, it actually is a key aspect in the cannabis plant, for medicinal purposes. Today, it's far applied in Cesamet (nabilone) and Marinol (dronabinol), via prescription.

How does medicinal marijuana artwork?

One of the maximum common questions most humans partner with medicinal marijuana is why ban the usage of marijuana at the same time as it's been positioned to have quite some blessings? Consequently, those people that question its use counter that there are one of a kind drugs that may be used which might be allowed legally so why bother with the use of an unlawful substance like marijuana?

Supporters of medicinal marijuana say that patients do no longer use marijuana in reality to revel in right or to get that distinct "immoderate". The laws exceeded in the states in which it is crook nation that marijuana can be used for medicinal capabilities. Proponents of medicinal marijuana counter that this hemp plant may be used correctly to ease signs and symptoms of positive clinical situations.

Key Ingredients and Medicinal Properties

The THC or tetrahydrocannabinol in marijuana is what offers clients the "excessive" feeling; however, it moreover brings cannabis severa its medicinal residences, including growing one's urge for meals. Your body clearly produces endocannabinoids, a substance that mimics the features of cannabinoids in marijuana. The endocannabinoid enables in regulating the frame's natural response to 1-of-a-kind stimuli. It is artificial handiest whilst needed but its effect is brief. There are endocannabinoid receptors located in the route of your body but they may be more first rate to your mind.

On the opportunity hand, the cannabinoids from marijuana bind the ones receptors, resulting to hundreds of medicinal blessings, which includes the bargain of pain and tension. Cannabinoids have additionally been determined to be a key substance inside the treatment of some styles of most cancers.

Today, there are artificial substitutes to marijuana that are allowed for medicinal use. However, most professionals say that those materials aren't as powerful due to the reality the real marijuana due to the reality there are compounds that can splendid be positioned within the cannabis plant which might be medically useful.

How Marijuana is Used?

Medicinal marijuana may be smoked, as with the normal workout of most customers. It also can be used as vapor; marijuana leaves are heated till all of the energetic additives are launched, but there can be no smoke formed within the path of this technique. Marijuana also may be eaten, as inside the form of sweet and cookies. It is also to be had as liquid extract.

Marijuana Use Relieves Chronic Pain

A current have a look at famous that a pant of marijuana a day helps relieve continual pain added about by using an damage or surgery. It moreover facilitates human beings sleep higher. Researchers located that the hashish plant relieves ache by using way of using changing the manner your nerves function. One of the principle advantages of hashish is to alleviate continual pain, however furthermore aids in palliative care and it efficiently enhances terrific pills, medicinal tablets, and remedy plans to assist treat high-quality medical conditions.

Understanding Chronic Pain

In continual pain, the indicators indicating pain are generated without physiologic importance. The signals are generated with out underlying reasons and the pain can often end up intense through the years. The herbal pain-relieving mechanism of the frame is deactivated. With everyday pain, there is a stimulus that triggers the ache as a manner to consequently elicit ache-relieving reaction.

The ache due to an damage or surgery is often accompanied with the aid of infection. Even if the damage heals, the ache remains, both it spreads to awesome elements of the body or it becomes chronic ache

Pain Components Likely to Respond to Marijuana

•Neuropathic components: the burning sensations

•Mechanical: the dull, pulsating, aching pain

•Inflammatory ache

Studies show that marijuana is able to assist within the remedy of a couple of pain syndromes, because of this hundreds of humans are gravitating towards the use of medicinal marijuana.

# Chapter 10: Pros And Cons Of Medicinal Marijuana

Researchers have diagnosed some of the feasible blessings and drawbacks of using marijuana as remedy:

•Marijuana is an terrific analgesic.

•There is a risk of mental addiction.

•Decrease in bodily dependence

•Minimal drug to drug interactions

•Tolerance to marijuana is in all likelihood to broaden

•For long time use, sufferers may want higher dosages

They have found in addition blessings to the use of medicinal marijuana, they embody the following:

•Excellent mood enhancer

•Spasticity

•Stimulates appetite

•Studies show that cannabinoids has neuro-defensive houses

•It is likewise anti-tumor impact

•There isn't any indication of breathing suppression

Studies show screen that the usage of marijuana can help patients suffering from the one of a kind types of chronic pain, along with the subsequent:

•MPS or Myofascial Pain Syndrome

•DN or Diabetic Neuropathy

•CPS or Central Pain Syndrome

•OA or Osteoarthritis

•RA or Rheumatoid Arthritis

•DP of Discogenic Back Pain

•PP or Phantom Pain

•NPS or Neuropathic Pain Syndrome

•MP or Malignant Pain

•SCI or Spinal Cord Injury

•HIV or HIV Neuropathy

There is a shape of chronic ache that has baffled scientific medical doctors, scientists, and researchers for years. FMS or Fibromyalgia Syndrome is not clean to deal with and there may be regardless of the truth that no recounted treatment for the infection as an awful lot as at the existing time. FMS causes debilitating ache even underneath treatment. With medicinal marijuana, there's desire for FMS patients.

The use of medicinal marijuana stays the hassle for debates. Medicinal marijuana in reality refers back to the raw product, which means the smoked form of the hashish plant. It isn't always similar to the synthesized shape of THC, that is an active substance in marijuana. Synthetic THC is one of the critical components for the anti-nausea drug, Marinol. It is prescribed especially to most cancers patients who're present gadget chemotherapy remedy. It changed into first authorized through the FDA in 1986 to ease chemo side results. A few years later after extra research and research completed, the enterprise authorized it for weight advantage specially for sufferers who've AIDS.

Is it Safe?

The US government, in its Controlled Substances Act of 1970, classified capsules and divided them into five businesses, referred to as schedules, based mostly on these three elements:

•Likelihood of triggering dependancy or abuse

•Medical advantages

•The dangers of physical and intellectual addiction

Is marijuana addictive?

A difficulty for lots customers is whether or not or no longer or now not they will turn out to be addicted. There are conflicting critiques concerning the addictive nature of marijuana. Recent research display that everywhere among 10 to 30% will make bigger dependency while handiest approximately 9% may also additionally have a critical dependancy. A large majority of clients by no means increase an dependancy and most humans can cease resultseasily.

Initially, marijuana become located, on the side of heroin and LSD underneath Schedule 1, which is the maximum addictive with little or no medicinal blessings. However, studies are beginning to trade the notion of the addictive potential of marijuana.

Minor Side Effects

So an awful lot has been said about the risks of marijuana and there are nevertheless some minor facet effects that aren't to be not noted, however they usually do now not closing very prolonged but it'll pay to be informed. These consist of:

•Drowsiness

•Dizziness

•Euphoria

•Memory loss

Anxiety and psychosis are located in a few clients due to prolonged dosage and substance abuse.

Limitations and Risks

Even if medicinal marijuana is crook in some states, it isn't always monitored with the resource of the FDA like all of the specific drug treatments that have met the approval necessities of the enterprise. The FDA has no facts about its potential damage in your health, or if it is a ability cancer cause.

Doctors wouldn't prescribe medicinal marijuana to everyone who's under 18 years of age. Patients who've been diagnosed with coronary coronary coronary heart illness and terrific coronary coronary coronary heart troubles are not allowed to use it as medicinal drug. If you're pregnant, it's also now not recommended.

Divulging your whole scientific statistics at the same time as you talk over with your clinical scientific medical doctor is crucial. Doctors will no longer prescribe medicinal marijuana to patients who have a information of psychosis.

## Chapter 11: Debunking Myths Of Medicinal Marijuana

A lot of things need to be taken into consideration in terms of using medicinal marijuana, even if you live in a rustic in which it's far legally allowed. People ought to be nicely-informed approximately the use of marijuana as medicine because of the dangers involved.

The Role of Pharmacists

•Aside from docs and researchers, pharmacists (and drug manufacturers) want to gather the duty in teaching patients on the right use of medicinal marijuana.

•It is also essential that they train and deliver counseling to the circle of relatives and the affected man or woman.

•It additionally may be a top notch issue if pharmacists might be involved in incorporating hashish to formulations to make ointments, medicinal pills, tinctures, and inhalers.

•They also can be useful in regulating the dosages.

•Because of their considerable records in pharmacology and tablets, they'll additionally be useful in ensuring that sufferers are given and using amazing immoderate excellent medicinal marijuana paperwork a amazing manner to beautify efficacy.

Debunking the Myths

If you want to comprehend if medicinal marijuana is for you, it's far vital to recognize greater about it. This phase discusses the specific famous myths approximately medicinal marijuana and some crucial information as a manner to debunk these myths.

Myth #1: Proponents to legalizing marijuana use for medicinal functions is just their manner of starting the doorways for the use of the substance for project.

The Facts:

•Experts have recognized the specific recuperation blessings of marijuana. Notwithstanding the dangers, they although advocate using medicinal marijuana to alleviate signs and signs and symptoms that encompass vomiting, nausea, and muscle spasticity.

•Several research have glad scientists that marijuana is an remarkable treatment. If conclusions approximately marijuana's recuperation homes had been now not based mostly on records, using THC will not be customary thru the FDA in manufacturing pills and capsules for some unique illnesses and clinical situations.

•Its right use an prolonged way outweighs the chance of abuse. With right training, guidance, and monitoring of patients, it could be an powerful ache reliever. The fact that a few mainstream and set up tablets can also be abused, marijuana should be considered for its efficacy inside the treatment of some ailments. Medicinal marijuana might not be too one-of-a-kind from medicinal capsules that also may be abused, like dozing tablets, anti-depressants, pain relievers, and tranquilizers.

Myth #2: Treatments other than marijuana are still higher.

The Facts:

•As with superb capsules, drug treatments, and remedies, humans reply in any other case. Because no people are the identical, it is expected that no people could have the identical reaction to treatments. An effective treatment for one person might not be suitable for each different. Likewise, one person may likely show off considered one of a kind factor consequences from a drug than those skilled through manner of every other. With exquisite frame compositions, ones frame can also react in any other manner to marijuana and other drugs.

•Your body has natural receptors for receiving cannabinoids. The chemical substances that serve the ones receptors are called anandamides. These anandamides are crucial for your frame's physiological make-up and features, in addition to control of motion, pain manipulate, memory retention, and motion manage. Marijuana is the only known natural deliver for cannabinoids and it's miles given to sufferers who cannot produce cannabinoids clearly.

Myth #3: The "marijuana tablet" is enough so different varieties of medicinal marijuana are no longer wished.

The Facts:

•THC has been authorized to be synthetically produced to be used as component in Marinol, a prescription drug. THC may additionally have medicinal benefits however marijuana's blessings are not derived completely from it. There are particular useful substances decided in marijuana that add to its medicinal performance.

•There are studies that show how powerful medicinal marijuana can be and some patients who can not get remedy from Marinol have determined it with medicinal marijuana. It is also important to point out that those sufferers who are displaying vomiting and nausea symptoms and symptoms discover it hard to swallow drugs and drugs; therefore marijuana is the favored choice.

•THC is actually the primary cause why marijuana may have toxic consequences on the human body. The specific lively substance in marijuana can help lessen its intoxicating consequences so sufferers who take the tablet are observed to be greater intoxicated than people who use marijuana. Dosage manage is much less tough with medicinal marijuana, too, because of the reality smoking has immediate consequences as compared to looking forward to the tablet to be digested and absorbed inside the body.

•Other factors in marijuana have extra restoration benefits than THC.

Myth #four: The legalization of marijuana for medicinal functions would probable have dire social outcomes.

The Facts:

•People want to be informed about legalizing marijuana for scientific use. For one, registration to this system is needed earlier than all people can plant and employ marijuana as medicinal drug. Should you take a look at in, you do no longer chance your fitness and your criminal and social fame.

•Those sufferers who will be producing their personal assets can be beneath safety and their identities stay guarded to prevent theft and first rate threats from unscrupulous human beings.

•For sufferers who do not have the functionality to supply or procure their personal materials, they are allowed to select out caregivers they take shipping of as proper with to cope with the purchase for them. The caregivers may additionally must be aware that any beside the component interest and unauthorized use of the affected person's medicinal marijuana has crook liabilities, no longer only for caregivers but additionally for the affected man or woman. There are software program hints that need to be accompanied with the beneficial aid of the patients, caregivers, and families.

Myth #five: The legalization of marijuana for medicinal capabilities can also make a one-of-a-type affect on the children.

The Facts:

• Pain medicinal drugs, tranquilizers, and morphine are more risky however they'll be being legally used as medicines. Youth aren't intended to use them as nicely however they've more get right of access to to them than marijuana.

Myth #6: It isn't always safe to legalize marijuana even for medicinal features because of the truth it is addictive.

The Facts:

• In studies done, marijuana can be considered as one of the most secure materials with restoration houses.

• There are only a few marijuana-related deaths in comparison to 1-of-a-type greater toxic tablets and materials.

## Chapter 12: A Simplified Look At Pain Killing Drugs

This financial disaster offers a simplified clarification of some of the important thing pharmaceutical capsules used to relieve pain. (The use of natural remedies complementary to these pills is described in Chapter 4.)

Complementary remedy is the utilization of each traditional remedy and opportunity-herbal tablets concurrently to gain a more steady and further effective remedy for the affected individual. Alternative-natural drugs may be brought to the treatment via the doctor to lessen the dosages of the pharmaceutical drug to keep away from undesirable factor outcomes inside the affected man or woman, or truely to growth the recuperation effectiveness of the treatment. Van Wyk and Wink (2010) described the usage of Stinging nettle (Urtica dioica) for its anti-inflammatory homes as a complement to that of non-steroidal anti inflammatory tablets (NSAIDs) in the remedy of arthritis. By which includes Stinging nettle to the treatment, the physician have become able to achieve greater anti inflammatory interest and keep away from elevating the dosage degree of the NSAID.

Other key healing additives of ache control, which include sleep, exercise and vitamins are not mentioned on this chapter. Since ache also can furthermore save you you from falling asleep or from having a restful sleep, your clinical medical doctor might also additionally prescribe pharmaceutical sleeping aids. Weight loss and exercising will also be part of the medical doctor's recovery software to help you get better. For instance, excessive body weight places plenty extra weight on a knee joint, and this more strain at the joint will make contributions to the degree of ache. Obesity is also a contributing detail to osteoarthritis due to the extra weight at the joints.

In the case of fibromyalgia, severa studies have proven that restful sleep is a key detail to the healing of the affected individual. Some of the research tested bargain in pain associated with patients obtaining restful sleep. It is likewise vital for sufferers with fibromyalgia to exercising regardless of the fatigue. Exercise brings multiple advantages to the affected man or woman starting from stimulating the immune gadget, relieving strain, stimulating the manufacturing of endorphins, to growing endurance. Exercising does no longer suggest turning into a professional athlete. It manner beginning with easy adjustments, which includes strolling for half-hour 3 days every week, or extraordinary slight workout at the facet of swimming, and with time slowly growing the depth and amount of exercise.

images

Note:

This monetary catastrophe provides some of the aspect consequences which may be said for the pharmaceutical drug. The reader desires to recognize that those single artificial molecules are typically powerful pharmacological sellers and have provided superb pain treatment to many patients. Some people are greater sensitive than others to the outcomes of those tablets, and others are virtually searching out a natural treatment. Many humans take these pharmaceutical drugs and do no longer revel in any of the aspect outcomes described underneath. In some times, humans to start with experience undesirable effects however, over time, their body turns into capable of way the drug and the element effects disappear. You need to communicate to your medical doctor about complementary remedy, if you are a affected character that memories some of the undesirable results of a drug.

images

Anti-inflammatory Remedies

These drugs are frequently used to help reduce ache and are normally known as Non-Steroidal Anti-Inflammatory Drugs (NSAIDs). Over-the-counter (OTC) NSAIDs embody aspirin and ibuprofen (Advil®, Motrin®). Prescription NSAIDs in Canada encompass naproxen (Naprosyn®) and celecoxib (Celebrex®). These capsules have been spherical for a extraordinarily long time but, in reality, have been round a very short time in comparison to a few natural treatments.

Anti-inflammatory herbs can reduce pain with the aid of reducing the infection. Inflammation of a tissue subsequent to harm or sickness can be without a doubt or in aspect liable for the pain. The mechanism of motion of NSAIDs is the inhibition of prostaglandins. Prostaglandins are worried in infection and ache. Some NSAIDs certainly have a non-prostaglandin mechanism of motion that contributes to its effectiveness. Sometimes you have a look at approximately capsules which is probably COX inhibitors. COX is the abbreviation for cyclooxygenase and this enzyme device is worried in the production of prostaglandins. COX-1 and COX-2 inhibitors are, consequently, capsules that act through the prostaglandin mechanism of movement.

NSAIDs may be effective in relieving infection and pain because of muscle pain, menstrual ache, headache, low lower back ache, arthritis,

Over the fast time period, those capsules by myself might also additionally moreover offer enough pain consolation, but the pain will go again if the situation isn't treated. Many times an anti inflammatory drug isn't always enough to triumph over the ache. The doctor can also additionally want to apply distinct drugs, which embody analgesics and muscle relaxants, or flip to unconventional tablets like antidepressants for pain alleviation.

171

When used on the advocated dosages and dose frequency, the ones anti inflammatory capsules can be effective pain killing medicinal tablets. Over-dose or long time use can bring about toxicity to the frame, which incorporates gastrointestinal harm (e.G. Dyspepsia, peptic ulcers, bleeding), renal toxicity (e.G. Acute renal failure, nephritic syndrome, worsening of high blood pressure), cardiovascular consequences (antiplatelet residences of aspirin, coronary risk) and hepatic harm. These pharmaceutical dealers are acknowledged to purpose toxicity even supposing used on the encouraged dosages. Some people are more susceptible than others. Sometimes it is the combination of medication taken in a day which could motive an interaction and ultimately toxicity.

Drug Quality

We have a tendency to nice fear approximately the awesome of herbal fitness products, but if we examine the facts releases during the last  years, we are able to in all likelihood be surprised to look the amount of ache killer over the counter (OTC) medicines recalled from the marketplace. These recollects have been associated with the awesome of the goods. The hassle blanketed contamination of the goods inside the course of manufacturing thru extraordinary factors. Be vigilant at the same time as buying OTC pain killers and visit Health Canada's internet web site that lists recalled pills:

1.     Visit the media room at Health Canada for the modern advisories and recollects at http://www.Hc-sc.Gc.Ca/ahc-asc/media/advisories-avis/index-eng.Php

2.     Visit the drug do not forget listing at Health Canada: http://www.Hc-sc.Gc.Ca/dhp-mps/compliconform/preserve in thoughts-retrait/_list/index-eng.Personal domestic page

Analgesic Remedies

When we pay attention of analgesics we both don't forget Tylenol®. Some humans additionally think of Motrin® as an analgesic. From a ache treatment thing of view, every are accurate due to the fact analgesia is defined due to the fact the discount or removal of ache. From a pharmacological aspect of view (e.G. Mechanism of motion on the body to reduce pain), the term analgesic is used to outline factors that act on a purpose within the body. Its motion is what offers us the sensation that the ache is reduced. In extraordinary words, the difficulty blocks or stops the sign of pain to the mind which usually translates this signal to inform us that it hurts.

Some of the pharmaceutical components relieve ache no longer via manner of manner of performing at the net web site of the frame's harm however with the resource of acting right now on our thoughts that translates this damage signal. Other pharmaceutical elements act proper now at the internet site online and save you the sign from going to the mind.

Acetaminophen (e.G. Tylenol®) has been spherical for the cause that early Nineteen Fifties and stays a amazing first preference analgesic. Patients should never take extra than 4 grams in step with day of acetaminophen. Acetaminophen is decided in each OTC and prescription ache medicines. Compared to many specific analgesics, acetaminophen has a super safety profile in terms of undesirable facet outcomes. Its maximum not unusual side effect is nausea. Acetaminophen may additionally cause liver toxicity even as overdoses are taken and, even as taken chronically, it can motive liver harm.

The United States Food and Drug Administration (FDA) has requested manufacturers of acetaminophen prescription merchandise (e.G.

Acetaminophen + hydrocodone (Lortab®)) to reduce the electricity of drugs and tablets to 325 mg in keeping with pill. Additional facts in this problem is available at: http://www.Fda.Gov/Drugs/DrugSafety/uc m239821.Htm. In addition, the FDA is forcing manufacturers to add a black container caution to the label of all prescription products containing acetaminophen bringing up that there can be a capability for excessive liver harm, and allergies (e.G. Swelling of the face, mouth, and throat, problem respiratory, itching, or rash). This alternate isn't always required for OTC acetaminophen merchandise, considering the fact that those warnings already appear at the label.

Unfortunately, many pharmaceutical drugs that act as analgesics have unwanted aspect consequences and plenty of moreover cause bodily dependence. Both of those homes appreciably restrict the doctor's capacity to relieve pain at the same time as maintaining the affected person's super of existence. Many parents have taken narcotics and bear in mind waking up the subsequent morning with hangover-like signs and symptoms. This is just one of the side consequences expert thru way of people taking opioid narcotics. Opioid narcotics are materials that act on opioid receptors in our frame and their motion on the receptor outcomes in blocking the signal of ache. The other aspect results of opioid narcotics range from ordinary dreams, agitation, aggression, apprehension, attention disturbances, impaired coordination, despair, confusion, cognitive ailment, dizziness, drowsiness, dysphoria, euphoria, hallucinations, headache, insomnia, bodily dependence, reminiscence impairment, temper adjustments, nervousness, panic attacks, and so on. A full listing of those is available out of your pharmacist.

Although the perception of getting the above aspect results sounds horrific, it is important to consider that they do offer pain comfort in conditions in which no particular stores are able to help the patient, specially in instances in which the ache is insufferable to the affected individual. When sellers have vital component results, it's far even more important to adhere to the guidelines made thru the scientific medical doctor and or pharmacist. Talk for your physician or pharmacist about any other tablets, or natural health merchandise, which you are taking, as those is probably elements that make you prone to getting some of those element results. Some herbal fitness merchandise, together with herbs, additionally can be a factor that makes you greater at risk of the consequences of a drug.

To some humans it's far surprising to pay attention that antidepressant medicinal pills are used as analgesics. In reality, a number of the ones pills have been used for decades to relieve pain particularly conditions like fibromyalgia, migraines, and neuropathies from diabetes. Some of the better antidepressants used embody tricyclic antidepressants (TCAs) (e.G. Amitriptyline®, Desipramine®), serotonin-selective reuptake inhibitors typically referred to as SSRIs (e.G. Paxil®), and selective serotonin and norepinephrine reuptake inhibitors (called SNRIs) (e.G. Cymbalta®). Clinical studies tested that those capsules may be effective analgesics at dosages lower than what's used to address situations like depression.

Although the efficacy of those pills in relieving ache may be right, their component effects regularly bring about the affected individual stopping the medication. In simple terms, preserve in mind that those pills were initially designed to act on the thoughts to help patients get over troubles like melancholy or obsessive compulsion. Simply, the ones pills act at the mind's chemistry to correct the imbalances which might be answerable for the ailment. Based in this primary hobby of the drug, it isn't sudden to locate that the difficulty outcomes in someone with out a neurological-related contamination, like depression, are unbearable. The real mechanism of movement for the pain consolation of antidepressants isn't regarded, but it in fact is a cease result of the medicine motion on dreams internal our brain or spinal wire (taken into consideration a part of the essential disturbing device).

TCAs established desirable efficacy at low dosages however patients can't tolerate the sturdy sedative and anticholinergic (e.G. Acts on nerves to reduce spasms of easy muscle organizations) consequences. Interestingly, the more current antidepressant medicinal capsules (e.G. SSRIs and SNRIs) are considered to have fewer component outcomes than the TCAs. Paxil®, an SSRI, which has medical trial proof of ache treatment, unluckily reasons insupportable factor consequences in plenty of sufferers however what pharmacologists idea. These aspect consequences embody anxiety, agitation, regular desires, impaired awareness, depersonalization, amnesia, confusion, muscle pain, muscle twitching, muscle vulnerable factor, joint ache, and so on.

In instances of intense ache, severa tablets can be given to obtain extra comfort. Some fitness professionals can also add an NSAID to the each day treatment with acetaminophen to similarly lessen ache. If the affected individual continues to be in ache, the expert can also then add a susceptible opioid appearing drug to try to lessen the ache. This pharmacological technique to ache remedy should best be achieved through manner of a fitness-care professional, as there are many implications to combining tablets, beginning from functionality drug-drug interactions to additive or synergistic outcomes, that could cease end result from the mixture.

Drugs that potentiate the ache remedy even as given in mixture with an analgesic are called adjuvant-analgesic capsules (e.G. Clonidine® it definitely is an alpha-2-adrenergic agonist). They are referred to as adjuvant analgesics, and now not as analgesics, due to the fact primarily based on its mechanism of movement the pharmaceutical producer did now not to begin with increase the drug for pain comfort.

Lyrica® is an analgesic and changed into the primary drug accepted for the remedy of fibromyalgia. It is a prescription analgesic that is significantly applied to address neuropathic ache. It moreover has detail effects that a few patients discover unwanted, at the facet of dizziness, ataxia, and so forth. In instances of excessive neuropathic pain, it can be combined with special ache killers, along side opioid narcotics.

Muscle Relaxant Drugs

The beauty of products called skeletal muscle relaxants (e.G. Flexeril®) is used to deal with muscle spasms related to painful musculoskeletal conditions. These tablets are frequently implemented in combination with analgesics to achieve pain alleviation. For instance, sufferers with L4 or L5 disc hernias also can additionally get episodes of immoderate muscle cramping of their decrease limbs. Flexeril® is normally used as a muscle relaxant to treat these muscle spasms.

The unwanted issue results of Flexeril® include drowsiness, dizziness, confusion, irritability, reduced intellectual acuity, skeletal muscle susceptible factor, and many others.

Other Drugs

Other pharmaceutical pills like benzodiazepines (e.G. Clonazepam®) are used to assist relieve ache. Benzodiazepines had been verified clinically to assist a few patients with fibromyalgia by means of the use of exciting demanding, painful muscle groups together with helping the affected person gather deep sleep.

Another magnificence of pharmaceutical drugs called alpha-2-adrenergic agonists (e.G. Clonidine®) offers ache remedy thru the usage of performing at three awesome websites: the mind, spinal twine and in peripheral tissues. This beauty of drugs is used for neuropathic ache.